BRAVING
CHEMO

BRAVING
CHEMO

WHAT TO EXPECT,
HOW TO PREPARE AND
HOW TO GET THROUGH IT

BEVERLY A. ZAVALETA, MD

Sugar Plum Press, LLC

To chemotherapy patients everywhere,
may you find courage.

CONTENTS

AUTHOR'S NOTE

*B*raving Chemo is a book about how to care for yourself in order to feel better while undergoing chemotherapy. This book is for you if:

- You have been diagnosed with cancer and will be starting chemotherapy, especially a very intense regimen.
- You are currently undergoing chemotherapy, especially a very intense regimen.
- You are caring for someone who is having chemotherapy and you want to learn more about what they are going through.
- You have a friend or loved one who is having chemotherapy and you want to give the book as a gift.

A *different* book would be better if:

- You are having immunotherapy but not traditional chemotherapy.
- You are having radiation and surgery but not chemotherapy.
- You are finished with chemotherapy and want a book that focuses on Cancer Survivorship—only chapter 7 of this book is about Recovery and Survivorship.

Remember that the information and suggestions in *Braving Chemo* are not meant to replace the advice of your oncologist or other doctors. Always attend your medical appointments, ask questions whenever you need clarification and get permission from your doctor before implementing the advice in this book and especially before starting any new medication or supplement. With this in mind, you can stay informed and work together with your oncologist to make chemotherapy as effective and comfortable as possible.

INTRODUCTION

Getting a cancer diagnosis feels like a bomb going off—in the doctor's exam room, in your brain and in your life. I got my cancer diagnosis news over the phone, since my family physician is also a personal friend. I had been standing in the middle of my son's end-of-school swimming party, loading drinks into a cooler with one hand while my other hand mashed the phone to my ear. When I heard the words "infiltrating ductal carcinoma," the most common type of breast cancer, time seemed to slow down. My friend Michelle, hostess of this up-to-now happy occasion, gazed at me with curiosity, then trailed after me as I strode like a zombie through her house and out the front door. I must have turned white, or maybe green, because once I choked out a few words, she said simply, "I'm here," and pulled me to her in a giant hug.

As a family physician, I had treated many patients with cancer and thought I understood their concerns and needs when they were going through chemotherapy. But after I found myself on the other side of a cancer diagnosis, I began to understand how much I had yet to learn. I thought I'd be able to continue working at least part time, as I'd urged many patients to do, but due to the intensity of my treatment, I was unable to see any patients or work at all. As time went on, I discovered that for all the challenges I faced as a patient, my training as a family physician and a hospitalist gave me insight that very few cancer patients have. On one hand, I knew immediately how aggressive my cancer was (scary!), but on the other hand, I was able to have detailed discussions with my oncologist about the newest treatment options available (reassuring!). I had my share of setbacks (collapsed lung!), but I used my professional knowledge to protect myself and tried to prevent side effects. Once the mental paralysis of getting a cancer diagnosis wore off, I got busy learning how to care for myself and how to accept help from family and friends.

I went through chemotherapy with a physician's understanding of the side effects, knowing what would happen to my body and why, what to expect and not to expect. If I had a question, I knew where to look to find the answer, and I could understand the explanation. Other cancer patients, however, who lacked my medical training and experience, were struggling to find answers to basic questions. Throughout my several months of chemotherapy treatment, several friends came to me with questions from their own family members who were undergoing chemotherapy during this same period. My friends expressed their loved ones' doubts about treatment, difficulties with side effects or questions about diet, and they asked for my help. Apparently, there were many people who felt that they lacked the information they needed to make informed decisions or take care of themselves.

But how could this be? After searching online and in person, I had discovered that there are numerous cancer-focused websites, apps, trackers, organizations, books and helplines. All this information is in addition to the "chemo class" given by a chemotherapy nurse that most oncologists require their patients to take before starting chemotherapy, as well as the various instruction handouts and information brochures that cancer centers give out. But despite these high-quality resources, I was listening to the stories of people who were struggling and suffering: my girlfriend's sister with breast cancer in Michigan, my neighbor's cousin with lymphoma in Iowa, the mother of my son's classmate with breast cancer. So it wasn't long before I found myself answering their questions, not in the medical office exam room, but over the phone or via email. As I recovered from my treatment, I continued to answer their chemo questions, and my own, and the compilation of these questions and answers became *Braving Chemo*.

Braving Chemo is a concise guide for cancer patients undergoing chemotherapy, providing answers to the common worries, problems and questions that arise during chemo. From what to take with you to treatment to how to hang in there when you feel like giving up, this book provides you with the answers and guidance you need at a time when your body, mind and spirit feel overwhelmed and making any decision at all can be a monumental feat. Even if you are not the patient but instead are the support person for someone having chemotherapy, this book will be a valuable resource for you to inform yourself about what your loved one needs to know during chemo.

We all have different learning styles and most people need to see or hear information more than once in order to remember it. Some people prefer to research a topic thoroughly and read in-depth, while other people would rather have a bulleted list of instructions. *Braving Chemo* isn't meant to replace the instructions that you get from your oncologist and chemo treatment team but rather to compliment and augment the advice. *Braving Chemo* is a convenient reference manual for you to have on hand at home, and together with the information from your oncologist, you can use the guidance in the book to make your chemotherapy treatment more effective and less unpleasant.

I have organized this book so that you won't need to read it cover-to-cover or in any particular order, since I know that you don't always have the time nor the stamina to do so. If you need to read it on and off, out of order, or return to parts of it again, that's okay. Each topic will stand on its own. If you read the book all the way through before you begin chemotherapy, that's great—you will be well prepared. If you read each section as it applies to where you are in your chemo treatment, that will work too.

Keep in mind as you read that not everything in the book will apply to you—you should always talk to your oncologist about how to apply the advice to your specific situation. This is especially true if you have advanced or metastatic cancer, or if you are on immunotherapy.

Immunotherapy is not the same as chemotherapy and has very different side effects. Finally, if you give this book to a loved one who is having chemo, consider reading it first to inform yourself about what lies ahead. Whenever and however you read *Braving Chemo*, I hope that you use it in the way you find works best for you.

I am learning that cancer recovery and survivorship is a continuous process. To help you in your own recovery process, the final chapters of the book are devoted to this topic of rediscovering and rebuilding your life after completing a course of chemotherapy. As scary as this challenge is, I am here with you to explore, to teach, to encourage and to remind you that you can be brave, even when you feel fearful. Thank you for allowing me to join you.

CHAPTER 1

GETTING STARTED

GET YOUR GAME ON

You are about to begin chemotherapy. You are in a serious competition—not with anyone else or for any material prize—but for your life. Your treatment stretches before you, as a physical, mental and spiritual challenge, not unlike a triathlon. I have stood at this starting line where you now stand, heart pounding, wishing to be anywhere else. The odds seem unfavorable, the rules bewildering and the physical demands terrifying. Your health is at stake, as is the chance to live your best life. And that means that you must break out of your stupor, rally your energy and get your game on. Here's a pregame warmup to get your head in the game:

> *Reach in.*
> *Reach deep into yourself.*
> *Find your reserves of energy, of courage, of life.*
> *Even if you cannot feel this energy now, it is already within you,*
> *Already there for when you will need it.*

As my own post-diagnosis shock slowly thawed, I realized this: in this cancer triathlon, I would have a game plan, coaches and teammates. There would be rest stops along the way. I learned over time that there would be surprise laughter and crazy moments of joy, not just stumbles or the pain of twisted ankles. That pounding of my heart became my drumbeat, leading me forward and keeping me in the game.

Allow your pounding heart to become your drumbeat, and that drumbeat will see you through this difficult, challenging time. No matter what you've been through in the past, no matter how new—or not so new—this health challenge is for you, you have what you need to compete in this personal triathlon, and you can prevail. So let's get started.

ACKNOWLEDGE YOUR FEAR

The thought of starting chemotherapy is terrifying to most people. The good news is modern chemotherapy drugs and the medications used along with them allow most people to do well, with far fewer side effects than in years past. Yet each person is different. Some will respond to chemotherapy with few debilitating side effects as they continue to work, take care of their families and live their lives nearly normally. Others may be wiped out, sick all the time and unable to do much more than get out of bed each morning and crawl back into it each night. But all will wonder, how will I feel? How will my body react? How will I know if the chemo is working? The uncertainty of not knowing what's up ahead, with the possibility of death looming, leaves everyone afraid.

Acknowledge your fear, and you will begin to find your courage. You don't have to understand exactly what you're afraid of—your fears may change over time. Right now, your fear might be of losing your hair or throwing up in the chemo chair. My fear was of dying while my children were still very young.

Whatever your fears, when you are ready, try acknowledging them with this exercise which will help you to do that.

Acknowledge Your Fear
Close your eyes and notice if you are afraid at this moment. Take a few long, slow breaths. If you sense fear, just let it be there.

Feel your heart beating by placing your hand on your chest if you need to. Keep breathing and stay with the fear, observing it.

Being brave does not mean that you have no fear; it means that you continue forward with your fear because what you are doing matters.

Notice that fear itself cannot hurt you.

You are safe and intact.

You are strong and whole.

Feel your heart beating, moving you forward.

Use this exercise whenever you feel overwhelmed. Even in a public place, no one has to know that you are doing it. Breathing requires no special equipment, and you don't have to lie down or sit in any specific posture. You can always breathe, acknowledge what is there and take a moment to let yourself settle. Now, if you are feeling a little braver, get ready to do some research.

WHY ASK WHY? THE IMPORTANCE OF QUESTIONS

So here you are, in the aftermath of the cancer bomb, having met with your oncologist and other members of your care team, ready to plan your treatment. No doubt you have been given some options, heard plenty of suggestions from well-meaning friends, and might be more confused than ever. Information overload is common. Fear and confusion are normal. But the more information you have, and the better you understand your options, the more confident you will be about your choices.

You will need to ask lots of questions, and the more information you have, the better your questions for your medical team can be. Don't rely on your oncologist or the chemo nursing staff to provide you all the answers—despite their best efforts, and they will be working very hard, they can't anticipate all your questions or read your mind. So, even if you feel overwhelmed by information, it's worth the effort to ask questions so that you can understand your treatment options.

Once you have a good understanding of your cancer and your treatment options, you will feel that you can make the correct choices for you. You will feel comfortable that the treatment you choose will match what you value for yourself and your life goals. For example, do you want the most aggressive treatment in order to obtain a cure, even if the side effects are more severe? Do you want to avoid surgery and choose other treatments instead if available? Do you want to choose a chemotherapy regimen that is longer but would allow you to keep working between treatments?

This is your chance to make sure that your game plan is right for you. To help you create that plan, the following section details strategies for working with your doctor and care team, as well as a list of websites and resources for doing your research. Gear up and investigate!

GATHER YOUR INFORMATION

Now that you understand why you must do the hard work of learning about your type of cancer and what type of treatment will be best for you, let's look at the strategies. First, *ask questions*. This may seem obvious, but it is actually very difficult. It's hard to know what you don't know, and difficult to remember what you wanted to ask when you are sitting in the doctor's exam room. So make a list of questions before each visit and bring it with you. Since you may have no idea what to ask, at the end of this section I've included a sample list of questions to get you started.

Bring a support person to your doctor visits, such as your partner or spouse, a friend or a family member. This way you will have two sets of ears to listen, and two minds to process the information. The stress of being told that you have cancer makes it difficult to hear, understand and remember all the information that your doctor tells you. A support person can help by writing down what the doctor says and asking questions that you might not think of.

Clarify exactly what type of cancer you have and how advanced it is. This includes the stage, grade and molecular or genetic subtypes. These characteristics will determine the treatment options that are available to you. Write down this information (or have your support person do so) so that when you research treatment options, you know that you are reading about treatments that apply to your specific type of cancer.

⬥ DEFINITION: MOLECULAR AND GENETIC MARKERS

Molecular tumor markers, also called genetic markers, are genes that are mutated or overactive in cancer cells. When drugs can be targeted to these mutated genes, or to the proteins that these genes produce, this is called "targeted therapy."

Some people find that creating a file and keeping copies of lab tests, radiology scans and biopsy reports is very helpful. You will need to bring this file of information with you if you get a second opinion.

Many types of cancer, such as lung cancer, are tested for gene mutations with specialized genetic testing panels, either through blood tests or testing on the tumor tissue. The results of genetic tests can influence what type of chemotherapy, or other treatments such as immunotherapy or "targeted therapy," will work for your cancer. Ask your oncologist if genetic testing and targeted therapy is available at your cancer center. If your oncologist does not offer genetic testing and targeted therapy, consider getting a second opinion at a larger cancer center. The National Cancer Institute, Office of Cancer Centers' website lists all the comprehensive cancer centers in the United States, and the resource list below can help you find a large cancer center near you.

🏷 DEFINITION: IMMUNOTHERAPY

Immunotherapy is a type of medical treatment for cancer, given either intravenously or taken orally, that activates the body's immune system to fight the cancer cells.

Read up on your type of cancer by going to a reputable cancer website, such as the sites listed below. You may want to compare the treatment regimen that your doctor suggests to the standard treatment for your specific cancer, such as the guidelines published by the American Society of Clinical Oncology (ASCO). However, note that some cancers do not have specified treatment guidelines, and treatment is very individualized. The cancer websites listed below describe typical treatments for different types of cancers.

Consider participating in a clinical research study. Research studies can be especially beneficial for people with advanced or rare cancers. Ask your oncologist if a research study would benefit you and is available to you through her office. The National Cancer Institute has a list of all clinical trials currently being conducted everywhere in the country, searchable by cancer type.

Make sure to discuss the treatment proposal with your family or support person. Someone who knows you well can help you make decisions when you are under stress. If you feel unsure, consider getting a second opinion about your treatment options, especially if you have an uncommon type of cancer or live in an area without a large, comprehensive cancer center. Finally, schedule another appointment with the oncologist to get all your questions answered before starting your treatment.

Questions to Ask Your Oncologist

1. What is the full name of my cancer?
2. What is the grade and stage of my cancer?
3. Is there a molecular/genetic subtype to my tumor? Are there any tumor markers? How does the tumor marker affect my treatment options?
4. Has my cancer spread beyond the primary tumor?
5. What are the different treatment plan options?
6. Other than chemotherapy, what other treatments will I need to have (such as radiation, immunotherapy, surgery or oral medications)?
7. Do I qualify for a clinical research study?
8. What are the side effects of the treatment that you are recommending?
9. How long will the total treatment last?
10. How long will it take to recover from the treatment side effects?
11. Will I be able to work (go to school, take care of my family) during this treatment?
12. Is the goal of this treatment to cure my cancer? If my cancer is not curable, what are the goals for controlling or suppressing my cancer?
13. In the case of late-stage cancer or advanced metastatic cancer: Am I a candidate for palliative care or a hospice program?

DEFINITION: PALLIATIVE CARE

Palliative care is specialized care for people living with a serious illness. The focus of palliative care is not on treating the disease, but instead on providing relief from pain and other symptoms. Palliative care regards dying as a normal process, integrates the psychological and spiritual aspects of patient care and offers a support system to help patients live as actively as possible until death.

You may want to bring this list of questions with you to the first several visits and revisit them. Sometimes the goals of treatment change, and sometimes the treatment plan changes as things move along. Keep asking questions, keep taking notes and keep researching. Use the resources below to help you.

The following websites and apps are reputable tools and sources of cancer information. Chemocare focuses only on chemotherapy, while other websites provide information of all sorts. The websites for the American Society of Clinical Oncology and the American Cancer Society are comprehensive and discuss everything from diagnosis and treatment to support and recovery. The apps listed provide help finding information as well as support resources. For people interested in finding a clinical research study, go to the websites for the National Cancer Institute or the National Institutes of Health.

Apps for Cancer Information and Treatment Navigation

- Breast Advocate at **https://breastadvocateapp.com/**
- Eva from Cancer Support Community at **https://eva-app.co/**
- NCCS Pocket Cancer Care Guide at
  https://www.canceradvocacy.org/resources/pocket-care-guide/
- This is Living with Cancer at
  https://www.thisislivingwithcancer.com/living-with-app

Website Resources for Cancer Information and Treatment Navigation

- American Cancer Society at https://www.cancer.org/
- American Society of Clinical Oncology at https://www.cancer.net/
- Cancer Care at https://www.cancercare.org/
- Cancer Council (Australia) at https://cancer.org.au/
- CareZone at https://carezone.com/home
- Chemocare from Cleveland Clinic at http://chemocare.com/
- Livestrong, a cancer support and resource organization at https://www.livestrong.org/
- Macmillan Cancer Support (United Kingdom) at https://www.macmillan.org.uk/
- National Cancer Institute at https://www.cancer.gov/
- National Cancer Institute, Office of Cancer Centers at https://cancercenters.cancer.gov/
- National Coalition for Cancer Survivorship at https://www.canceradvocacy.org/resources/pocket-care-guide/
- US Library of Medicine, National Institutes of Health (Pubmed) at https://www.ncbi.nlm.nih.gov/pubmed

PLAN FOR FERTILITY

Many types of chemotherapy can damage your body's reproductive system. For women, chemotherapy can shut down the ovaries, either temporarily or permanently. If the ovaries stop functioning permanently, a woman enters menopause and no longer ovulates or becomes pregnant without medical assistance. For men, chemotherapy can destroy the ability of the testicles to produce healthy sperm.

If you are of reproductive age and think you will want to have children after chemotherapy is finished, ask your oncologist about how your chemotherapy regimen will affect your fertility. If your chemo regimen typically causes infertility, discuss options to preserve your fertility before beginning chemotherapy. For men, fertility preservation means sperm banking, and this is almost always possible before starting chemotherapy. Ask your oncologist to refer you to a fertility specialist or a urologist to set up sperm banking before starting chemotherapy.

For women, there are various options for fertility preservation. If there is enough time, ovarian stimulation followed by egg retrieval and storage, or embryo storage, is a good option. In some cases, such as acute leukemias, there may not be enough time to perform these procedures before treatment must be started. Instead, women can undergo hormone suppression therapy with injections of a gonadotropin-releasing hormone (GnRH) analog, such as leuprolide (Lupron). Injections of GnRH analog shut down ovarian function during chemotherapy, and studies have shown that women with breast cancer who receive GnRH analog injections during chemotherapy have an improved chance of ovarian recovery after chemo is finished. It is unclear from the research whether treatment with GnRH analog preserves ovarian function in all cancers, but it's worth it to ask your doctor about this option. If preserving fertility is something that you are concerned about, ask for a referral to an oncofertility specialist.

The following resources are reliable sources of information about fertility planning before and after chemotherapy. The Oncofertility Consortium is a multi-specialty medical group at Northwestern University in Chicago and can be reached by the telephone hotline or on its website.

Oncofertility Resources

- The Oncofertility Consortium at Northwestern University, Chicago at **https://oncofertility.northwestern.edu/** or call 1-866-708-FERT
- *Huffington Post* article "Five Things You Should Know About Oncofertility" at **https://www.huffpost.com/entry/5-things-you-should-know-about-oncofertility_b_8037942?guccounter=1**
- Livestrong, a cancer support and resource organization at **https://www.livestrong.org/we-can-help/livestrong-fertility**

FIND YOUR MINDSET

The most common cancer mindset that you are likely to hear is the Battle. People often say things like, "He's battling cancer," and companies sell T-shirts that say, "Fight for the Cure." For some of us, this battle talk is what we need to get energized and ready. The fighting words give us courage. But when I was diagnosed, the Battle mindset made me feel unsettled. I wondered, if the cancer is part of me, then who exactly am I fighting—myself? Moreover, fighting a battle felt angry and violent, and I wanted to heal, not fight.

> ### ◈ DEFINITION: MINDSET
>
> A mindset is a mental attitude or inclination. It acts like a filter through which we see the world and interpret events. It even affects how we view our own feelings. Our mindset biases how we approach life.

Another common cancer mindset you may encounter is the Journey. There are numerous blogs and memoirs by cancer patients and survivors that tell their personal journeys of cancer treatment and recovery. These narratives describe the survivors' stories, the good and the bad of what they experienced with cancer, how they coped and what they learned. The Journey mindset is geared more toward approaching cancer and its treatment as a process of personal development. This approach can help you be open to learning from your experience of cancer and channeling your energy into growth opportunities. There is even an organization called The Cancer Journey (**https://www.thecancerjourney.com**) that trains accredited "cancer coaches," professionals who assist patients through the process of treatment and recovery. For some of us, this is the perfect approach. For others, the Journey mindset may strike us as rather whimsical, over-analytical or avoidant of the harsh realities of cancer. What to do?

There is no one correct cancer mindset. Each of us finds our own right path. On a good day I landed somewhere between the Battle and the Journey—in a mindset I envisioned as the Challenge, something more like a triathlon or a mountain climb. When I felt drained and in need of help, I found a Healing mindset to be more helpful. Putting it together, I tried to envision the physical, mental and spiritual challenges of chemo as part of doing the hard work of healing. Confronting cancer and going through chemo with a balance of a Challenge and Healing mindset required both grit and gentleness. Grit to keep me going even when I was scared or in pain, and gentleness to allow for recuperation and reflection when that was what I required. Because of this balance, I could acknowledge the horror of cancer but eventually continue to experience the beauty of living.

What is your mindset? Try the exercise below to practice different mindsets and see what feels right for you.

Finding Your Cancer Mindset

Visualize yourself on a Journey, winding your way step by step along a path. Slowly you pick your way forward, listening to your surroundings and your internal signals. What are you learning about yourself and about what matters to you? Can you see a goal ahead? Who is with you on this Journey? What does your best life look like?

- *Now try on a Battle Mindset. Visualize yourself as a powerful warrior standing tall. Sound the ancient battle cry: Come and Take It! Fighting words will help you feel brave. See yourself conquering cancer, with chemotherapy as a powerful weapon.*
- *How about a Challenge Mindset, such as training for a triathlon? Visualize yourself rising to the Challenge and winning the race. Be aware of how amazing and intelligent your body is! Have faith that your body knows how to heal and recover, with just this little nudge from chemo. Just like training for a*

competition, when you sleep, eat and focus your mind, you are preparing and maintaining your body for the physical stress of chemotherapy. You are capable of turning yourself into a chemo triathlon-winning machine!

- *Settle in to a Healing Mindset. Imagine your body gathering its resources, your cells renewing themselves, cleansing themselves from the inside out. Think of this healing state like hibernation, from which you will emerge refreshed and replenished. Allow the healing process to occur without much guidance from your thinking brain—your body knows how to do this!*

Finding your mindset is an important step toward facing cancer each day when you are undergoing chemotherapy. After you've done this exercise, you should have a better sense of the mindset that works best for you. You may find that more than one mindset works best at different points in your treatment! Remember to lean on the support that you have from family and friends—their love will keep you strong and help you through the tough parts. But in order for them to support you, you first must do something very difficult: tell them that you have cancer.

TALK TO YOUR PEOPLE

Telling your loved ones that you have cancer or are starting chemotherapy can feel worse than just having cancer. It's as if speaking of it makes it more real or more terrible. In the moment before you tell someone, you dread the pain that you will cause by revealing this awful thing. I almost couldn't bear telling my mother that I had been diagnosed with cancer—all I could think of was how sad or scared she might feel. Being a mother myself, I imagined the horror of my own children having cancer—or even worse, I imagined dying and leaving them motherless. At the time of my diagnosis, even though I was the one who needed caring for, I was wrapped up in worrying about others' reactions.

As much as you dread it, however, chemotherapy is happening, and eventually you need to tell people—people you trust. But here's the thing: who you tell, how much you tell them and when you tell them are all up to you. Telling the story takes energy, and your energy is precious. You need energy right now for thinking and planning. So if you need to take time to digest the news, tell no one at first or only your spouse or partner. Put off telling anyone else until you are ready. Stay on the couch for a week watching movies if you need to, before you decide your next move.

❤ HELPFUL HINT

Do not prematurely post on social media because cyberspace can be unforgiving. Once you post, it's hard to take it back—you may realize that you didn't want everyone to know everything. Plan how you want to use social media, and it can be a great resource for connecting you to far away family or to a cancer support community.

That being said, if you keep this cancer to yourself, you will become isolated. The fastest way off the island of isolation is to tell your closest family and friends that you have cancer and that you will be treated with chemotherapy. Your loved ones can be a source of energy and support. Let them be there for you. When I was diagnosed, I knew I would need the support of the people who loved me and the understanding of those who needed me. Like ripping off a bandage, I got it all over within 24 hours by calling my siblings, parents and ten close friends. I wanted my village notified.

TALK TO THE KIDS

Even more terrifying than telling your friends that you have cancer is talking to your children about having chemotherapy. If you have young children, you're likely wondering, will I be cracking their world apart? Will they break? When my husband and I sat down to tell our young boys about my cancer diagnosis and the plan for chemo, the moments leading up to saying the words felt surreal. There was a sense of finality, of destroying life as we knew it. Irrationally, I felt that by holding in the words I could prevent it from happening.

But of course, it was happening, and I realized that the kids wouldn't break. Kids are smart and tough. They need honesty and openness, and they need to continue to feel our love. Be straightforward, and if they're young, tell them something straightforward that explains the process to them, such as:

"I had a biopsy. That's a sample of body tissue, a test on a piece of the body that the doctor took out. The biopsy showed cancer—that's a disease that can be bad sometimes. It's a disease where the body cells go crazy and grow out of control.

"The doctors have discussed it, and they have a plan for some very strong medicine that should kill all those crazy cells. I'm going to get this medicine every few weeks through a tube that goes into my vein.

"Sometimes I'm going to be tired and not feel good. I might throw up. Sometimes I won't be able to leave the house. After a few weeks, my hair will fall out. But my body is very strong, and it knows how to heal itself with help from the medicine. My heart is very strong and brave. I need lots of hugs from you and that will help me feel better."

> ❤ **HELPFUL HINT**
>
> Find tips, conversation starters and many other resources and links at the website for Cancer Support Community at https://www.cancersupport-community.org/talking-kids-teens-about-cancer.

Teens and older children may want a more detailed explanation, and it's recommended to answer their questions as honestly and directly as possible. They may ask things like "Are you dying?" or "Will I get this too?" Consider bringing your child to meet your oncologist and ask if your cancer center has counseling available to the families of patients.

Let children know that it's normal to feel sad, scared or angry about cancer, and that it's fine to cry about it. Also, it's okay for your children to see you cry or be afraid. Feeling sad or scared about things that *are* sad or scary is normal. Showing your child that you can cry or feel scared while still continuing on is the definition of courage. Being brave in the face of fear may be one of the most valuable lessons that you can show to your children and to yourself.

GATHER YOUR GEAR

Getting into that chemo chair for the first time might feel like the most terrifying thing you have ever done. I felt like I had signed up to voluntarily step in front of a wrecking ball once a week. But you can make it a little easier by getting prepared. You will feel more relaxed and confident about doing well during chemotherapy if you have what you need before you start.

There are certain supplies that you will need at each chemo session, as well as a stock of items at home for recovery. For example, at home you'll need all your prescription medications filled and ready ahead of time, as well as foods and snacks that don't require lots of preparation. Prescription anti-nausea medications are a necessity to have on hand at home, and many people like to bring a chemo bag stocked with hard candies to suck on, a pillow and personal care items such as moisturizing eye drops and tissues. The two lists below, the Master Shopping List and the Chemo Day Packing List, include many of the things that you will need to take care of yourself during and after chemo. The Master Shopping List includes everything on the Chemo Day Packing List, as well as items that you will need at home over the next several weeks and months of your chemo treatment.

As you read over these lists, the purpose of certain items might seem unclear right now. The need for each item, how to use the items and all relevant details are explained in the next several chapters. For example, you will learn details on prevention and control of side effects, nutrition tips, facts about exercise during chemo and how to take care of your mental health. Feel free to skip ahead if you have a pressing problem right now, such as insomnia or constipation. Otherwise, be reassured that you will have all the information that you need by the time you get to the end of the book. Now, get shopping!

CHEMO MASTER SHOPPING LIST

Food and Drink

- Bottled water (many people find tap water nauseating)
- Variety of drinks, such as herbal teas, juices (pasteurized only), sports drinks, soda
- Protein drinks (such as Boost, Ensure, Glucerna, Atkin's Plus Protein)
- High-protein snacks (peanut butter, peanut butter crackers, granola bars, cheese sticks, yogurt, hummus, protein bars and shakes, protein powder for adding to smoothies)
- Ginger products such as tea, hard candies and chews (to combat nausea)
- Vinegar (for disinfecting vegetables/fruits, needed when immune system is low)

Miscellaneous Supplies & Equipment

- Small cooler or thermal bag (for bringing snacks or lunch to chemo)
- Throw blanket or wrap (you may frequently be cold)
- Entertainment: magazines, books, e-Reader, music/video player with headphones, laptop
- Soft hat or beanie to wear to bed (a hairless head can get cold)
- Wig, head scarves and hats (headwear for hair loss)
- Soft socks, sweatpants, loungewear (comfortable clothing for chemo)

Body Products

- Hand sanitizer, alcohol-based
- Moisturizing body cream, preferably unscented and paraben-free (Aveeno, Burt's Bees, CeraVe, Curel, Kiss My Face, Lubriderm, Nivea)
- Lip balm
- Lubricating eye drops, non-medicated, such as Systane or Refresh
- Saline nasal spray, non-medicated
- Mouth/oral rinse, moisturizing and alcohol-free, such as Biotene or MetaQil
- Soft toothbrush
- Facial tissues, boxes and pocket packs
- Oral thermometer, digital read

Medications

- Prescription medications from your doctor (for pain, nausea, constipation, anxiety, sleep). Fill all prescriptions in advance.
- Miralax powder (polyethylene glycol)—for constipation
- Dulcolax tablets (bisacodyl)—for constipation
- Senokot-S (senna concentrates)—for constipation
- Imodium (loperamide)—for diarrhea
- Pepto-Bismol (bismuth subsalicylate)—for diarrhea
- Diaper rash/skin barrier cream with zinc—for hemorrhoids or irritation

> **⚠ MEDICAL ALERT**
>
> For the over-the-counter medications listed above, review them with your doctor or care team, and make sure which ones are safe *for you* during chemotherapy.

- Tucks pads (witch hazel)—for hemorrhoids
- Tylenol (acetaminophen)—for pain and fever
- Tums (calcium carbonate)—antacid, for heartburn
- Zantac (ranitidine)—antacid, for heartburn
- Glutamine powder—an amino acid, to avoid mouth sores, nerve damage and diarrhea
- Melatonin—1mg and 3mg tablets, a naturally-occurring brain hormone, for insomnia
- Multivitamins and other vitamins per physician's orders

IT'S CHEMO DAY!

Now that you have all the supplies that you need for the long haul, you need to pack for the day of chemo. Usually, chemo infusions take several hours so bringing your own snacks and drinks is a good idea. In addition, most people have less nausea if they eat a light meal on the morning of chemo instead of starting on an empty stomach.

Chemotherapy rooms are typically cold due to air-conditioning, so it's a good idea to bring a sweater or blanket. It can also get boring, so think about what you want to do for entertainment: Watch a movie? Read? Take a nap? Make sure that your mobile devices are charged the night before and bring your chargers. Bring your own pillow if you think you will take a nap. Use the packing list below as a guide.

Chemo Day Packing List

- Medical insurance card, photo ID, money, credit cards
- Mobile phone and charger
- Hard candy or gum, such as mint or ginger (for taste distortion and nausea control)
- Cooler with drinks and high-protein snacks
- Water bottle
- Facial tissues (runny nose and watery eyes are common)
- Hand cream and lip balm (for dry skin and lips)
- Pillow and blanket (for taking a nap)
- Jacket or sweater, warm hat, warm socks or slippers (the chemo room is cold)
- Electronic device with headphones and charger (for entertainment such as listening to music or podcasts or watching movies)
- Reading material, such as magazines, books or an e-reader
- Activities, such as a coloring book, cards, knitting or crossword puzzles

- Prayer beads, prayer shawls, Bible or other spiritual reading
- Your chemo companion or a ride home—hard to "pack" but needed just the same!

After you have had a few rounds of treatment, you will figure out what you need to be comfortable. Most people find that eating a light meal the morning of chemo helps to avoid nausea, but you might find that it's better for you to avoid food before your treatment and just snack during the infusion. You may realize that you sleep most of the time and have no need for that bag of books you've been meaning to read! You may savor the three hours of uninterrupted movie-watching time, or you may look forward to catching up with a friend while your chemo is running. However you do it, gather your gear and you're ready.

BRING A BUDDY

It may help you to have someone keep you company during your chemotherapy infusions, especially at the beginning. Invite a companion who is comforting, supportive and nonjudgmental. You want to be relaxed, not worried about feeling embarrassed or vulnerable. If you like conversation, bring someone chatty . . . if you like quiet, bring someone who will sit and read while you take a nap.

There can also be camaraderie in the chemo room since sharing stories, or snacks, with other patients can lift your spirits and make you feel less alone. This is also a good time for your caregiver to meet other caregivers and swap information. Frequently, the bonds formed with other patients receiving chemotherapy on the same schedule turn into lifelong friendships.

> ❤ **HELPFUL HINT**
>
> If you don't have a good support system, help is available through groups such as the American Cancer Society, Cancer Support Community (https://www.mylifeline.org/), or Catholic Charities USA.

Some people prefer to be alone during their chemo infusions, and if you find that this is the case for you, don't be shy about declining any company. However, you should consider accepting a ride back and forth to all treatments, since you may be tired, nauseous or dizzy after treatment. It's a good idea to accept offers from different people to take you to treatment so that one helper doesn't get burned out. As with all things, follow your instincts regarding social time or alone time during your infusions so that you can be as relaxed and comfortable as possible.

BEFRIEND YOUR MEDICINE

It may seem impossible right now, but if you can see your chemotherapy treatment as a positive force helping you heal, you will be opening the door for the chemo to work together with your immune system to kill the cancer cells. You may be filled with fear or worry about the chemotherapy being toxic. You may doubt that you are strong enough to get through it. But by befriending your chemo, you can see it as your partner helping you to regain your health.

Visualization, a process of imagining and seeing in your mind's eye something that you want to make a reality, can help. To prepare yourself and create a friendly attitude toward your chemotherapy, try the following visualization exercise:

Befriend Your Medicine

Close your eyes and imagine the medicine flowing through your body, destroying the cancer cells. If you can, visualize the actual organ where the medicine is working.

Take a few long, slow breaths and imagine the cells of your immune system detecting and then killing the cancer cells.

Imagine your healthy cells staying healthy and each heartbeat delivering nutrients through your bloodstream to your healthy cells.

Feel how your body works to heal you, integrated and coordinated with the chemotherapy.

You can repeat this exercise again during your chemo infusion and afterwards when you are home. The chemo will be working in your body, and your body will be working with the chemo. Like giving yourself a mental hug, use this visualization whenever you want to give your chemo and your immune system a boost.

ACCEPT HELP

❤ **HELPFUL HINT**

Use your list of helpers and create a "call schedule" of who to call for daily assistance or emergencies. You can create a calendar of assigned activities based on the helpers' availability.

Coordinating doctor visits, receiving chemotherapy and recovering from each treatment cycle takes a tremendous amount of time and energy. Meanwhile, the rest of your life still has to function! This is true whether you are a household of one or raising a houseful of kids. Bills must be paid, meals have to be cooked and toilets have to be cleaned. On many days you will be too tired to do these things. Asking for help is essential to the daily running of your household during cancer treatment, and most of us are not good at asking for and receiving help. As a physician accustomed to caring for other people, I was terrible at asking for help. But on the day that I received my diagnosis, I realized that I could not survive this challenge alone. As my friends began to offer help with the kids or meals, I accepted. I urge you to do the same. Now is the time to reach out to your family and friends. You need to assemble the team of people who will support you and your family.

If you are married or in a relationship, your spouse or partner is usually at the top of the helper list. In addition to giving you love and emotional support, your partner may bear the brunt of the increased workload that chemotherapy adds to your life. To alleviate some of this partner overwork, create a list of people who are available to help, together with their contact info and availability. Once the people around you know that you are going through chemotherapy, you will be amazed at how they step forward to assist. What can be difficult is allowing yourself to accept the help and assigning them something specific that they can do.

The more specific you are about what you and your family need, the easier it is for people to help. Make lists of tasks that need to be done. Sort the task list into what you must do, and what can be done by someone else. Does your house need cleaning? Are you too ill to leave the house and need someone to run an errand for you? These are examples of tasks that someone else can do for you. Use the list below to get you started on delegating tasks to your team of helpers.

Tasks to Be Delegated

- Keeping your extended family and friends updated about your cancer (good task for a spouse or partner)
- House cleaning, especially toilets and garbage handling
- Laundry, ironing and dry cleaning
- Meal planning and grocery shopping
- Cooking
- Walking the dog, cleaning the cat litter box and other pet care duties
- Driving you to medical appointments
- Driving the kids to school or activities
- Shopping and other errands
- Yard and garden work
- Paying household bills
- Handling health insurance claims and bills
- Taking your spouse or children on an outing
- Helping you organize all these tasks!

Don't feel guilty about asking for help and receiving it. Remember that those who love you feel helpless right now, and they will be grateful for a chance to do something for you. Helping you is the physical manifestation of their love for you. Let them help and their love will carry you forward.

Resources for Accepting Help and Delegating Tasks

- Assistance & Care Organization Calendar at
  https://www.carecalendar.org//
- Cancer Council (Australia) at **https://cancer.org.au/**
- Cancer Support Community at
  https://www.cancersupportcommunity.org/
- Calendar templates in Microsoft Word at
  https://www.wincalendar.com/Calendar-and-Schedule-Templates
- Macmillan Cancer Support (United Kingdom) at
  https://www.macmillan.org.uk/
- Meal Organization Calendar at **https://www.mealtrain.com/**
- MyLifeLine at **https://www.mylifeline.org/**
- Nextdoor neighborhood organizer at **https://nextdoor.com/**
- Robin Care patient navigator service, available through some
  employers at **https://robincare.com/**
- Signup Genius at **https://www.signupgenius.com/**

WHAT TO DO ABOUT WORK

Getting your chemotherapy arranged and started takes time and it is hard work. It takes work to learn about your treatment options, to read, to think, to discuss, to pray, to prepare and to schedule.

Then there is your actual work—as in, what you do to make a living. Unless you are retired, you'll likely have to work. Whether you are a plumber, an executive, an entrepreneur, a teacher or a stay-at-home parent, you have a job and you need to figure out if you can, or should, keep working during chemotherapy. Some people work through most of their chemo, while some are totally disabled and don't work at all. Most people take intermittent time off and work when they feel well enough. Continuing to work at least part time usually helps people feel "normal" and more like themselves. Take some time to think about what will be best for you, based on your doctor's recommendations and your financial situation.

PROTECT YOUR INCOME

Planning carefully can help you keep working during chemotherapy. Know the laws in your state, province and country so that you can understand your rights. Here are some tips to help you protect your job and your income.

If you live in the US and you work at a large company, you may have benefits such as sick leave (or paid time off), short-term disability and long-term disability. If your company qualifies, federal law in the United States entitles you to 12 weeks of unpaid medical leave under the Family and Medical Leave Act (FMLA). While you are on FMLA leave, you cannot be fired from your job. You and your doctor will need to complete the necessary FMLA forms, however, and they are available from the US Department of Labor website. Forms for any company-specific paid time off or disability can be obtained from the human resources department. Laws in other countries vary greatly and you should refer to national employment websites.

Pause and think carefully before you tell your boss or employer any medical details, however. Disclosing medical information is not required by law. It is unfortunate but true that some employers discriminate because of medical conditions and your job could be at risk if you reveal your health condition. Only discuss your treatment plan with your boss and coworkers if they are supportive and if disclosing your illness will help you work out a flexible work arrangement, such as working from home or working alternative hours. Remember that sick leave and disability can be taken intermittently, and disability can be complete or partial (working part time). Taking partial disability can help extend your benefits out over a longer time, protect your job and help you keep working during treatment.

Visit your state's employment regulations website, as well as the FMLA website, to learn about your rights. The Young Survival Coalition, a group focused on young women diagnosed with breast cancer, has an excellent website (**https://youngsurvival.org**) that discusses cancer-related employment issues. This website has a comprehensive list of resources that are relevant to patients of all ages, with any type of cancer. The Cancer Legal Resource center is a non-profit organization that champions the civil rights of people with disabilities, including those with cancer. The website has extensive resources, including a downloadable handbook. Use the list of resources below to research your rights regarding working and employment during and after cancer treatment.

Resources for Employment Rights and Disability Leave

- Americans with Disabilities Act at **https://www.ada.gov/**
- Cancer and Careers at **https://www.cancerandcareers.org/en**
- Cancer Council (Australia) at **https://www.cancer.org.au/**
- Cancer Legal Resource Center at **https://thedrlc.org/cancer/**
- Cancer and Work (Canada) at **https://www.cancerandwork.ca/**
- Family and Medical Leave Act at **https://www.dol.gov/whd/fmla/index.htm**
- Genetic Information Nondiscrimination Act (2008) at **https://www.eeoc.gov//laws/statutes/gina.cfm**
- Macmillan Cancer Support (United Kingdom) at **https://www.macmillan.org.uk/information-and-support/organising/work-and-cancer**
- US Department of Labor at **https://www.dol.gov/general/topic/benefits-leave/fmla**
- Working with Cancer (United Kingdom) at **https://www.workingwithcancer.co.uk/**
- Young Survival Coalition at **https://www.youngsurvival.org/learn/living-with-breast-cancer/practical-concerns/careers**

ACKNOWLEDGE YOUR STRESS

Stress is part of daily life. All of us intuitively understand what ordinary stress looks like: juggling family schedules, getting bills paid, meeting work deadlines and coping with family conflicts. Often even good things are stressful, like getting married, being promoted or attending a family reunion. When I was diagnosed, I was halfway through packing up our house for a move, the kids had just gotten out for summer vacation and my extended family was scheduled to arrive for a visit. That was my everyday stress.

But cancer is different. Chemo is different. It's traumatic to hear that you have cancer and are facing chemotherapy treatment. Cancer can be life-threatening, and chemotherapy causes real suffering. When I was faced with an aggressive cancer and scheduled for chemo the following week, my stress went from the mundane stresses over moving and entertaining to worrying about if I would be fired from my job, thinking about side effects and fearing I might die. I was terrified.

So what happens when chemotherapy is added into the mix of our lives that are already stressful enough? Our stress skyrockets. Daily life continues regardless of the chemo calendar. We don't get to take a sabbatical from the ordinary—most things happening in life before cancer will still be happening. Despite the tremendous stress of starting my chemotherapy, I had to find a way to take care of myself and keep life going, without letting the stress consume me. My chemo calendar was set, and so was our moving date. Packing transformed from sorting and downsizing to throwing everything into boxes before the move-out deadline. We found help with the move, help with the kids and we got to my first chemo. Over time, I realized that finding ways to reduce, redirect or harness stress is the key to getting through chemotherapy while still living your life.

First, some clarification. What exactly is stress? Is it always bad? As mentioned above, we instinctively understand *stress* as a thing or situation that is difficult for us and feels unpleasant. However, stress can also be defined as our experience of an external circumstance, not the external circumstance itself. In other words, stress is an emotion or physical feeling that we have when something threatening occurs or we are in an uncomfortable situation—even if that situation is a positive one, such as throwing a party or planning a wedding. The stress that we feel can be big or small, routine or extraordinary. Our bodies respond to stressful situations in several ways, described by scientists over the last hundred years as the "stress response."

The most well-known stress response is a physical and emotional state known as the "fight-or-flight" response, also called the threat response. When we are exposed to something that we think is stressful or threatening, the threat response is triggered in the body. Our heart rate and blood pressure increase, the blood flow to our muscles increases, and our mental vigilance is heightened. This physical response is mediated by release of specific hormones, such as cortisol, testosterone, dehydro-epiandrosterone (DHEA) and adrenaline, which give us greater strength and stamina when we need it most. The threat response has helped humans survive since prehistoric times by keeping us alert, focused and ready to face potential dangers.

Do you recognize this threat response? I do. Before my first visit with my medical oncologist, I spent ten minutes outside her office, sitting in my car with my heart pounding, trying not to vomit. Was I alert to danger? Oh, yes. I was hyper-alert to a danger that my prehistoric brain thought was coming at me from whatever the oncologist was about to tell me. This wasn't exactly a helpful response, but it was me being my fully human self.

It is important to know that the threat response is a normal response to danger. It helps us to react and protect ourselves and others. And, as you will see below, this state of heart-pounding adrenaline high can be used to your advantage if you can learn *how* to use it.

When you live with an ongoing stressful circumstance, such as undergoing chemotherapy for cancer treatment, you risk having a constantly activated threat response. This isn't helpful or healthy, since studies show that living in a prolonged state of threat can cause many different health problems, such as high blood pressure, elevated blood sugar, suppressed immune system function and increased inflammation. According to the latest research, what drives this increased risk of illness seems to be the chronically high levels of the stress hormones cortisol and adrenaline, coupled with high levels of fear and anxiety that occur during a threat response. Even for people without cancer, this is not a healthy state for mind or body.

So what can we do when faced with the extreme stress of cancer and chemotherapy? Advice to reduce our stress doesn't really make sense, since we don't have a choice in the matter. Did you choose to get cancer? I didn't think so. Fortunately, new scientific research about stress shows some fascinating and helpful findings. As stated previously, there is a difference between events and situations in our environment that place stress on us and the way that we feel about or respond to these events.

> ♥ **HELPFUL HINT**
>
> Even when you cannot control a situation, you can choose how to respond.

Dr. Kelly McGonigal is a Stanford researcher, professor of psychology and a leading expert on stress. She defines stress the following way: "Stress arises when something you care about is at stake." In other words, *stress* is something that we feel and experience in response to something happening around us. Dr. McGonigal has written and lectured extensively on the last several years of new stress research showing that there are numerous ways that we can respond when we feel stressed.

Recent research shows that stress is not inherently bad for us when we approach it from the right frame of mind. Several studies have shown that when people can see benefits of a stressful situation, such as seeing it as an opportunity for growth, they are more likely to respond to the stress with coping strategies that are helpful and healthy. The research on stress has described several responses to stress that allow people to weather stressful situations well. The good news is, you can train your-self to see the potential benefits of stress and to respond to stress in ways other than the classic threat response, in ways that are more beneficial and adaptive. In the next section, I describe these responses and hope-fully expand the way that you think about stress—and maybe show you how to use it to your advantage.

TRANSFORM YOUR STRESS

You're already aware that you are confronting something exceptionally stressful: chemotherapy. Maybe you are feeling *stressed*. Is your heart pounding? Palms sweaty and stomach churning? If so, your brain has triggered the threat stress response and right now being in that state won't do you much good. The threat response serves us best when it can save us from an immediate physical danger, such as escaping from an attacker or stopping a child from running into traffic. The threat response is a state of physical and mental high alert, and, as you now know, living in a state of constant high alert can damage your body and lead to problems such as insomnia and a low immune system. Plus, it's miserable! But stressful situations are part of life, and according to new research, stress does make us stronger if we respond in the right manner.

As described by Dr. Kelly McGonigal in her book, *The Upside of Stress*, you can transform your stress response into something more useful and helpful. The book provides a detailed look at the research and how it applies to improving our responses to stress. Below, I summarize what you need to know while facing the stress of chemotherapy.

⚠ **MEDICAL ALERT**

If you are feeling so stressed out that you can't sleep or are having trouble functioning, ask your doctor to evaluate you for depression and anxiety. Sometimes medications are needed to treat these conditions.

First, realize that you have a choice about how you respond to stressful circumstances. Recent research has discovered that there are at least three other ways that humans respond to stressful situations: by rising to the challenge, by learning and growing, and by connecting to others for support. Rising to the challenge means facing the stressful situation and engaging with it while feeling empowered. The challenge response is similar to the threat response in that we feel our hearts pounding, our blood racing and our senses heightened. But instead of feeling anxious, fearful and small, we feel tall. Instead of cowed, we feel confident. The hormones of the stress response are activated, but this time in an adaptive, healthy and functional way. When we feel challenged instead of threatened, we clearly see the cause of our stress and we step up to the plate. We may still feel fear but are not paralyzed by it. We feel that we have the resources to handle the situation, and we are motivated to do so.

A growth response is another way that we can harness the energy of something stressful. This response to stress takes a stressful situation and sees opportunity for learning and development. You may recall this idea from the Journey mindset that I discussed earlier. Research has shown that when people are able to find and create meaning in their experiences, even traumatic experiences, they are happier and healthier in the following years. This is not to say that meaning must be found in everything or that "everything happens for a reason"—it doesn't. Loss, death, illness and other such things are tragic and painful, and no one should force false positivity upon them. I would never say that I'm glad that I had cancer so that I could write this book, or that the *reason* that I had cancer was so that I would write this book. However, I *did* have cancer and I'm glad that I've been able to write this book and hopefully help others who are struggling with chemotherapy. There is a subtle difference.

> ❤ **HELPFUL HINT**
>
> Don't force yourself to try to find meaning in the midst of tragedy. Instead, be open to the possibility that, perhaps in time, there may be something good that grows out of what you are experiencing. This doesn't erase your pain or anger but co-exists with it.

Through my experience of having cancer and cancer treatment, I've gained a more profound insight into the suffering of patients and of how severe illness affects people's lives. I was humbled to learn that, despite my best efforts and intentions, my previous understanding and concern for patients was, in fact, somewhat superficial. Now I find that my compassion for patients has been multiplied exponentially. This is a breathtaking surprise and it gives me a small spark of joy in the aftermath of a traumatic experience.

A third adaptive and healthy response to stress is connecting to others for support. In this response, we reach out to those around us for help instead of isolating ourselves when feeling stressed. This could mean asking for the advice of others, seeking the physical closeness of our loved ones or reaching out on social media. This connection response is particularly helpful when we recognize that a problem is larger than ourselves and that we will need the resources of other people to get through it. These resources could be time, knowledge or actual material things such as food, money or transportation. For some people, this type of stress response, called the "tend and befriend response" by Dr. McGonigal, is second nature. For others, connection needs to be practiced in order to feel natural.

The existence of these beneficial stress responses is not just theoretical or observed solely in human behavior, but also has been shown by measurements of specific combinations of hormones. The levels and combinations of hormones that are present during a connection response, growth response or a challenge response are different than those in the threat response. For example, in all stress responses, cortisol and adrenaline are released, but levels of testosterone are higher during both the challenge and growth responses as compared to the threat response. Oxytocin levels are higher during a connection response and dehydroepiandrosterone (DHEA) levels are higher during a growth response. While the details and consequences of these hormonal differences are quite complex, the general gist is that oxytocin promotes feeling connected to one another, and DHEA promotes neuron growth and learning. Most significantly, DHEA and oxytocin are not associated with the long-term poor health effects that are seen with a prolonged threat state, and neither are cortisol and adrenaline if you have testosterone on board, such as during a challenge state! What the science shows is that when you learn new responses to stress, you are learning a way to turn stress into a tool to make you stronger, smarter and more connected to humanity!

Certainly, you should use whatever steps you can to reduce sources of stress. For example, many of the organizational strategies in this book don't just keep you organized—they are also intended to reduce sources of stress! However, given that stress is inevitable, I encourage you to reframe the way you think of stress—even this great stress of chemotherapy—and as Dr. Kelly McGonigal says, learn to "get better at stress!" Harness and transform your stress response first by using exercise, mindfulness and other relaxation practices to reduce your threat response, and then you can begin to enter a challenge response, growth response or connection response. You will feel more relaxed, prepared and supported. Your feelings of fear and anxiety will decrease, and you will be ready to strategize, learn, reach out for support and face the challenge. Even as you confront chemotherapy, you will be strong and brave.

Revisit Your Cancer Mindset
- *What cancer mindset have you been using, Battle, Journey, Healing or Challenge? These mindsets can help you harness a helpful stress response.*
- *If you have a Journey Mindset, then you are harnessing the Growth Response. Keep learning and finding meaning as you experience your treatment.*
- *A Healing Mindset is harnessing the Growth Response and the Connection Response to forge helpful connections both within yourself and within your support community.*
- *If you are in a Battle or Challenge Mindset, then this is the Challenge Response. Keep gathering your resources, pumping yourself up for the hard work ahead and feeling confident and powerful.*

- *Regardless of cancer mindset, you can always use the Connection Response by reaching out to your village of loved ones to gather support. Even when this is hard because you are feeling tired or shy, the payoff is huge. When you need help, a hug or just some company, let someone know.*
- *If you still feel in your gut that stress is always harmful, don't force it! It's hard to change a longtime habit and hard to take a positive view of something that feels bad. Try to make room in your mind for curiosity: What can I learn from this?*

BEFRIEND YOUR STRESS

As previously mentioned, the first step to harnessing the energy of this stressful time is to turn your threat response into a challenge, growth or connection response. To do this, you first have to calm the threat response—that is, you have to relax. Once your head is a bit clearer, you will be better able to see things as they are—and perhaps to accept the negatives and appreciate the positives. Then you can use the energy that stress gives you and turn it into motivation and determination, which will sustain you through this time.

Calming the threat response can be very difficult, given how many books, classes and therapies exist that specialize in "stress reduction." If you have a preferred way to relax and soothe yourself when you feel stressed, now is the time to practice this regularly. If not, this list is a quick reminder of things we can do to relieve feelings of stress.

Calming the Threat Response

- Listen to music
- Take a bath or shower
- Hug a loved one
- Take a walk
- Do breath exercises, meditation or prayer
- Snuggle your pet
- Practice a creative hobby— drawing or painting (try an adult coloring book!), baking, knitting, Lego building
- Sing or play an instrument
- Be outside in nature—work in the garden, walk in a forest or park, sit by a lake or the ocean

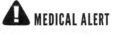 MEDICAL ALERT

It can be tempting to have a cocktail to relax, but drinking alcohol or using drugs (other than prescribed) is especially harmful during chemotherapy. Alcohol also interferes with sleep and can make insomnia worse.

- Get physical exercise—walking, biking, paddle boarding, dancing
- Laugh—listen to a funny podcast or watch a comedy

A wonderful exercise for experiencing a profound and connected embrace with your loved one is the Three-Breath Hug. This exercise was described by the global spiritual teacher, Vietnamese Zen master Thich Nhat Hanh. A prolific teacher and author, Thich Nhat Hanh is a worldwide leader of mindfulness and meditation, as well as a poet and peace activist. Try the Three-Breath Hug exercise below to improve your hugging skills and deepen your connection to others.

Three-Breath Hug

Embrace a loved one to start your hug. Breathe in slowly, then breathe out slowly. Settle into the hug, relaxing your shoulders and letting go of any tightness. During the second in-breath, fully feel the hug. Focus on the feeling of your arms and chests connecting. Notice how your breathing is synchronized as you breathe out. Breathe in slowly for the third breath, then release the hug after your third out-breath.

"When you hold a child in your arms, or hug your mother or husband, or your friend, if you breathe in and out three times, your happiness will be multiplied at least tenfold."

—Thich Nhat Hanh

BE GENTLE WITH YOURSELF

Remember that chemotherapy is a tremendous challenge. Be gentle with yourself and temper your expectations. Realize that your usual routine will change, and that's just fine for now. Say no to projects and parties. Save your energy for you, for healing and recovering. Sleep more when you need to, talk less when you need to and allow others to help you.

This challenge will not last forever, but right now listen to what your body is telling you. You will hear what is best for you. Today and every day, you can guide yourself gently and bravely.

CHAPTER 2

PREVENTING AND TREATING SIDE EFFECTS

P oison. This is what comes to mind for many people when they hear the word chemotherapy. The fear of side effects, such as vomiting and hair loss, can be so great that I have seen patients refuse chemotherapy just to avoid its side effects—even when the benefits of chemo would have been tremendous. This is unfortunate because modern chemotherapy is generally less toxic than older regimens and, with the correct knowledge, many of the side effects are avoidable or treatable. No one should avoid chemotherapy because of side effects or fear of side effects.

Of course, it is absolutely critical that each person weigh the risks and benefits of the proposed treatment plan, including the possible side effects. However, in my medical practice, I've seen that it can be extremely difficult for patients to understand the risks and benefits of a proposed treatment. When it comes to understanding and managing the side effects of chemotherapy, this is even more difficult because the stakes are so high. As a patient, I've lived the experience of managing chemo's side effects. I was fortunate to be able to apply my medical knowledge to what was happening to my body and put that together with my oncologist's instructions to come up with a strategy that could keep me as healthy as possible and get me through treatment.

This chapter is all about those strategies for preventing as many side effects as possible and treating the ones that do come along. I review many common side effects of chemotherapy and discuss how to prevent and manage them. These side effects include unpleasant things like hair loss, taste distortion, nausea, peripheral neuropathy (nerve damage) and constipation. By knowing what to expect, you can keep yourself as healthy as possible during chemotherapy treatment and keep your chemo treatments on schedule. Preventing side effects will not only prevent treatment delays but it will also make you feel better and make your chemotherapy as effective as possible.

IS BALD BEAUTIFUL? HAIR LOSS

No one dies of hair loss. Also called alopecia, hair loss from chemotherapy may be the most dreaded of all side effects. The thought of having clumps of hair fall out in the shower or waking up with hair on your pillow is particularly horrifying to some people. Seeing your own bald head in the mirror day after day reminds you that you are not yourself. Being bald can be an unbearable daily reminder of having cancer.

A bald head is also an outward sign of cancer. When I was finally hairless after a month of chemo, I got the sense that when people looked at me, even though I was wearing a head scarf, they saw the face of death. Confronting cancer isn't for the faint of heart, and your bald head will get right up in people's faces. You will find out who can handle it and who will avoid their own discomfort by avoiding you.

But there is good news: losing your hair is not necessarily required as part of chemo! First, several modern chemotherapy regimens, such as that for colon cancer, *do not cause hair loss*. Ask your doctor if hair loss is expected from your particular chemotherapy regimen. Second, there is a new treatment, called scalp hypothermia, that can prevent hair loss during chemotherapy if started at your first chemo treatment.

Scalp hypothermia, commonly known as "cold cap" treatment, is an FDA-approved process that reduces the hair loss from chemotherapy by cooling the scalp with a specialized device worn on the head during chemotherapy. Scalp cooling reduces the blood flow to the scalp, which reduces the amount of chemo drug that the scalp receives. This, in turn, reduces the toxic effects of the chemotherapy on the hair follicles and reduces the amount of hair that falls out by about 30–50 percent.

> ♥ **HELPFUL HINT**
>
> Visit the website for The Rapunzel Project (https://www.rapunzelproject.org), a non-profit organization dedicated to helping chemotherapy patients keep their hair during treatment.

There are several systems for scalp hypothermia available on the market, which are listed below. The equipment is usually rented, and private health insurance plans may cover some of the cost. If you can't afford to rent the equipment, visit **https://www.rapunzelproject.org** for assistance with obtaining a cold cap setup.

If preventing hair loss is important to you, plan to use scalp hypothermia. But be aware that *in order for scalp hypothermia to be effective at preventing hair loss, you need to start it at your first chemo treatment.* If you plan on going the traditional route of wearing a wig, hat or head scarf to cover your hairless head, then don't fuss with cold cap scalp treatment, and watch for more tips about head scarves, wigs and hats later in the book.

Hair Loss Prevention Resources

- Chemo Cold Caps at **https://chemocoldcaps.com/**
- Paxman at **https://www.paxmanusa.com/**
- Penguin Cold Caps at **https://penguincoldcaps.com/us/**
- The Rapunzel Project at **https://rapunzelproject.org/**

HAIR LOSS HURTS: WHAT TO DO WHEN IT STARTS TO FALL

Losing your hair hurts—literally hurts. Your scalp will be sore as the hair falls out of the follicles. Not only does it physically hurt, but for some, going bald marks the moment when there is no more denying the reality of having cancer. There is nothing like seeing your bald head in the mirror every morning to drive that point home.

Many patients, both men and women, choose to cut their hair in a shorter style in preparation for chemo. If your chemo regimen will cause you to lose your hair, consider whether wearing a shorter haircut might ease your emotional transition to bald. Another benefit of a haircut is that shorter hair puts less weight on your hair follicles, which causes less physical pain as your hair falls out.

> ❤️ **HELPFUL HINT**
>
> If you plan to wear a wig, research and order your wig as soon as you start chemo-therapy. If you plan to use a cold cap to prevent hair loss, order it before you begin chemotherapy.

Whether or not you are using a cold cap to retain hair during chemo, you may want to try to prolong the time that you keep your hair. Try these tips for minimizing discomfort and maintaining your hair as long as possible.

Tips to Retain Hair During Chemo Hair Loss

- Cut hair to a short style to put less weight on the hair follicles
- Shampoo gently and only every other day
- Style wet hair with a wide-toothed comb
- Avoid using a brush
- Avoid pulling on your hair during drying or styling
- Use only light-weight style products or none at all

At some point you will have patches of remaining hair. You can use electric clippers set to the closest setting to shave off these remaining patches or shave with a razor and shaving cream. Some hair salons will offer scalp shaves to chemo patients free of charge. After you shave, massage your scalp with a gentle skin toner containing witch hazel, and then apply a scalp oil. This soothes the scalp and helps to release stubble. If your scalp is dry, massage in a small amount of a natural body oil such as almond oil, coconut oil or an unscented body moisturizer.

♥ **HELPFUL HINT**

For information on scalp cryotherapy to keep your hair during chemo, visit The Rapunzel Project (https://www.rapunzelproject.org), a non-profit organization dedicated to helping chemotherapy patients keep their hair during treatment.

METAL MOUTH: TASTE DISTORTION

Feel like you are sucking on a penny? Distortion of taste and smell is a common side effect of chemotherapy. Many patients describe having a constant metallic taste in their mouth or the sensation of a burned tongue. These effects of chemo on the taste buds, nerves and brain can distort the taste of food and dampen your appetite. Sometimes taste distortion starts right during the first treatment, and it can last for several weeks or months after the last chemo treatment is over. Try the tricks listed below to reduce metallic taste.

Metallic Taste Tips

- Suck on hard candies or lozenges, or chew gum. Strong flavors such as mint and ginger work especially well for some people.
- Put a lozenge in your mouth before you receive any intravenous "flush" or chemo infusion through your IV catheter. This will counteract the rush of bad taste that some people get when the catheter is flushed.
- Rinse your mouth frequently with an alcohol-free mouth rinse, such as Biotene or MetaQil.

⚠ **MEDICAL ALERT**

During chemo, do not use mouthwash that contains alcohol since alcohol can irritate the mouth, worsen soreness or cause ulcers.

FIRE BREATHER: MOUTH SORES AND MUCOSITIS

Sometimes the damage that chemo causes inside your mouth is more than just a bad taste. If that bite of pasta with marinara sauce goes down like a hot coal, you probably have mucositis caused by chemotherapy. Mouth sores, ulcers and irritation are all types of mucositis. Mucositis can occur in the lining of the mouth, throat and esophagus, and symptoms include pain with chewing and swallowing, changes in taste and dry mouth. Symptoms can start the day of treatment or several days afterwards. Mucositis is caused by decreased saliva production during chemo, as well as by direct toxic effects of the medications on the lining of the mouth and throat. Try these strategies below to keep your mouth in good shape.

Preventing and Treating Chemo Mucositis

- Take glutamine powder supplement, 15g twice daily, mixed with a drink, pudding, ice cream or yogurt. Glutamine powder is available at health food stores or online.
- Suck on ice chips during chemotherapy infusion. This reduces the blood flow and amount of chemo medicine delivered to the lining of your mouth and reduces the toxic effect.

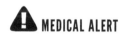 **MEDICAL ALERT**

Xylitol is very toxic to pets, so keep products containing xylitol out of reach of pets.

- Avoid any mouthwash containing alcohol.
- Use a mouth rinse containing xylitol, such as Biotene, twice daily or more, and chew gum containing xylitol.
- Do not use a tongue scraper—it will traumatize your tongue.
- Use only a very soft toothbrush and toothpaste made for sensitive teeth and gums.

- Avoid acidic foods (such as citrus and tomato), spicy foods and hot temperature foods for a few days after your treatment.
- To treat ulcers and pain, rinse your mouth with a mixture of equal parts Mylanta and liquid Benadryl. Swish, gargle and spit every three hours.
- If you have severe pain, ask your doctor for a prescription mouth rinse called "Pink Magic," which contains Mylanta, Benadryl and viscous lidocaine (a topical anesthetic).

♥ **HELPFUL HINT**

To treat mouth sores, take glutamine powder supplement, 15g twice daily, mixed with a drink, pudding, ice cream or yogurt. Glutamine powder is available at health food stores or online.

Swish, gargle and spit every three hours and before every meal.
- Ask your doctor to check you for thrush. Thrush is a painful yeast infection of the mouth and esophagus that can occur when your immune system is low, such as during chemotherapy. Thrush is treated with prescription antifungal medications.
- Try "oil pulling" to soothe your mouth. Swish two teaspoons of cooking-grade coconut oil in your mouth for up to two minutes, then spit.

If you have moderate to severe mucositis, it will be hard to chew and painful to swallow. If you can't swallow, you can't eat. If you can't eat, you can't take in enough food and fluids, and you won't get the fuel that you need to stay strong and heal. However, prevention and treatment of mucositis is possible—with a little diligence you will be able to keep yourself well.

⚠ **MEDICAL ALERT**

Ask your doctor before starting any type of vitamin or supplement.

FEET ON FIRE: NEUROPATHY

Many chemotherapy medications can cause a type of nerve damage called chemotherapy-induced peripheral neuropathy, or CIPN. Neuropathy symptoms are numbness, tingling, pain and weakness in your toes, feet, legs, fingers and hands. The symptoms usually start after several doses of chemotherapy and may be mild at first, affecting just the toes and fingers. Pain and numbness then progress up the feet, legs and hands. Severe neuropathy symptoms can impair balance, walking and doing daily activities.

Neuropathy can also begin or worsen after chemotherapy is over because the chemo medications are still present in your body for weeks to months. This is also true because nerve endings that were damaged by chemo slowly cease to function after chemo treatment is finished. Studies show that between 40–60 percent of chemotherapy patients have neuropathy at some point during or after treatment. Neuropathy is usually reversible, but some patients have permanent residual nerve damage and symptoms.

⚠ MEDICAL ALERT

If you have any of the neuropathy symptoms listed here, tell your oncologist immediately. Your oncologist should start you on a treatment for the neuropathy or might reduce your chemotherapy dose.

Chemotherapy Drugs that Frequently Cause Neuropathy

- 5-fluorouracil/5-FU
- Epothilones (Ixempra/ixabepilone)
- Hexamethylmelamin/HMM
- Platinum Analogs (carboplatin, cisplatin, oxaliplatin)
- Proteasome inhibitors
- Taxanes (Taxol/Onxol/paclitaxel, Taxotere/Docefrez/docetaxel, Abraxane/paclitaxel, Jevtana/cabazitaxel)
- Thalidomide
- Vinca Alkaloids (vincristine, vinblastine, vinorelbine)

Neuropathy Prevention

Unfortunately, there *is no medication, treatment or natural supplement that has been definitively shown to prevent chemotherapy-induced peripheral neuropathy*. For this reason, if you start to have symptoms of peripheral neuropathy, you should discuss the symptoms with your oncologist immediately. Your oncologist will monitor your symptoms and, in some cases, reduce the dose of your chemotherapy. In addition to chemo dose reduction, there is some research evidence that shows that cryotherapy using frozen gel mitts and booties to cool your hands and feet while you're receiving your chemo may be effective for preventing CIPN. For example, studies have shown that cooling mitts and booties used for patients receiving taxanes, a class of chemotherapy drugs, reduced the risk and severity of CIPN. Ask your doctor about using cooling mitts and booties during chemo infusions if you are receiving a taxane drug.

Research has been conducted on several natural supplements and other interventions, such as exercise, for CIPN prevention. The list below shows the interventions that are most promising according to the initial results. Keep in mind that the scientific evidence showing that these interventions are effective is still minimal.

Interventions to Prevent Neuropathy

- Frozen cooling gel mitts/booties, worn during each chemotherapy infusion
- Glutamine powder, 15g orally twice daily
- Vitamin B6, 150mg orally twice daily
- Omega-3 fatty acids (DHA/ALA), 1000–2000mg orally once daily
- Exercise, during and after chemotherapy

> **⚠ MEDICAL ALERT**
>
> Always ask your doctor before starting any new medication or supplement.

Neuropathy Treatment

Once symptoms of CIPN have started, the most effective treatment for chemotherapy-induced neuropathy is the prescription medication duloxetine (Cymbalta). Duloxetine is safe to take both during and after chemotherapy and is recommended for improving the symptoms of neuropathy by ASCO, the American Society of Clinical Oncology. There is also research evidence that shows that exercise and acupuncture improve neuropathy. Exercise and acupuncture can be done both while your chemo is ongoing and continued when chemo is finished.

According to research, the following supplements show some effectiveness for treating CIPN: acetyl-L-carnitine, alpha lipoic acid, curcumin, green tea extract, melatonin and omega-3 fatty acids. Only melatonin and omega-3 fatty acids (fish oil) are safe to take if you are still undergoing chemo—the

> **♥ HELPFUL HINT**
>
> The most effective treatment for CIPN (chemotherapy-induced peripheral neuropathy) is duloxetine (Cymbalta). This prescription medication is recommended by ASCO, the American Society of Clinical Oncology.

rest could interfere with chemotherapy and you should not take them unless chemo is over. Studies have also shown what *does not* work: vitamin E, and the prescription medications gabapentin (Neurontin) and pregabalin (Lyrica). These medicines are effective for other types of neuropathy, such as diabetic neuropathy, but are not effective treatments for chemotherapy-induced neuropathy.

Neuropathy Treatments Safe Both During and After Chemo

- Acupuncture
- Cooling mitts/booties
- Duloxetine (Cymbalta) prescription medication (cannot be taken with tamoxifen)
- Exercise
- Glutamine powder, 15g twice daily
- Melatonin, 3–30mg at bedtime
- Omega-3 fatty acids (DHA/ALA), 1000–2000mg daily
- Vitamin B6, 150mg twice daily
- Vitamin D, 2000–5000 IU daily (requires monitoring of blood levels)

Neuropathy Treatments Safe Only After Chemo

- Alpha lipoic acid, 600mg three times daily
- Curcumin, 500mg twice daily
- Green tea extract, 250mg daily
- Acetyl-L-carnitine, 500–750mg, twice daily

Nerves can heal, but they heal slowly, at most about one inch per month. For

⚠ **MEDICAL ALERT**

Many supplements are not safe to take if you are still receiving chemotherapy. Ask your doctor before starting any type of vitamin or supplement.

most people, this means a minimum of six–twelve months to heal neuropathy, and frequently longer. Give a new medication at least four weeks to see results and a new supplement at least eight weeks before switching. For acupuncture, a typical course is six weekly sessions.

❤ **HELPFUL HINT**

Try acupuncture for neuropathy! The most recent research shows that acupuncture improves peripheral neuropathy caused by chemotherapy—both reducing pain and improving function.

Do as much as you can, but balance activity and rest. Elevate your feet when you need to, and try massage or using tingly foot cream. Apply warm packs or ice packs, whichever feels better. Protect your feet in supportive shoes and boots with good insoles. Keep your oncologist updated about your neuropathy symptoms and, if possible, be patient.

WORSHIPPING THE PORCELAIN GODDESS: NAUSEA AND VOMITING

Second only to hair loss, nausea and vomiting are often what people fear most about having chemotherapy. Even the thought of nausea can make you nauseated. However, with preparation, you can prevent most nausea and vomiting.

Take comfort in knowing that at the start of each chemo treatment infusion, you will get intravenous medications to prevent nausea, such as diphenhydramine (Benadryl), palonosetron (Aloxi) and dexamethasone. These drugs are heavy hitters. They are much stronger than medications of years ago, and the anti-nausea effect lasts for several hours. Most patients feel fine during the chemo treatment, without any nausea.

In addition to the anti-nausea medications that you will receive through the IV line, your doctor will prescribe anti-nausea medication for you to take during the days following each chemo treatment. Don't wait until you're nauseated to have the prescriptions filled—fill them as soon as you get them! The list below shows a few of the most commonly prescribed anti-nausea medications that your oncologist may give you to have on hand at home.

> ❤ **HELPFUL HINT**
>
> If you have a long distance to travel to and from chemotherapy, take your nausea medication with you to treatment.

Common Anti-Nausea Medications

- Granisetron transdermal (Sancuso)—patch, apply the day before treatment
- Ondansetron (Zofran)—tablet, orally dissolving tablet
- Prochlorperazine (Compazine)—tablet, rectal suppository
- Promethazine (Phenergan)—tablet, rectal suppository, topical gel
- Steroids (dexamethasone, prednisone, methylprednisolone)—tablets

Finally, heartburn can also cause nausea. Have an over-the-counter antacid on hand such as calcium carbonate (Tums), aluminum/magnesium hydroxide (Maalox or Mylanta), ranitidine (Zantac) or famotidine (Pepcid).

STAY ON A SCHEDULE: TAKE YOUR NAUSEA MEDICATION

As described in the previous section, modern pre-chemo medications to prevent nausea are great. But do not be caught by surprise when the IV medication wears off—take your first anti-nausea pill a few hours after your chemo treatment finishes. If you are traveling or staying overnight away from home, make sure that you bring your medicines with you.

Take anti-nausea medication on a schedule for the first 24–48 hours after each chemotherapy treatment. Staying on a schedule helps you to stay ahead of the game. Remember, it's important to prevent nausea from progressing to vomiting that prevents you from eating and drinking.

> ❤ **HELPFUL HINT**
>
> Do not wait until you are nauseated to take anti-nausea medication—take the first anti-nausea pill a few hours after chemotherapy, even if you still feel fine.

There is no shame in taking medication to prevent nausea. There is no need to "tough it out." This will only cause you unnecessary suffering. Preventing and treating nausea will help you heal faster, so treat yourself kindly and take your medication.

TIME TO EAT: AVOID HUNGER TO PREVENT NAUSEA

Keeping food in your stomach will help prevent nausea. Eat a light meal the morning of chemotherapy treatment, unless specifically instructed not to by your doctor, and take a few snacks with you to chemo so that you have some food on hand. Popular snacks include crackers, granola bars, energy drinks and fruit.

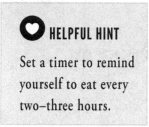

HELPFUL HINT

Set a timer to remind yourself to eat every two–three hours.

After you get home from treatment, eat a small meal or snack every two–three hours. Remember that an empty stomach will make you feel even more nauseous! Stay well-hydrated by sipping on liquids such as water, tea, broth or sports drinks. Experiment with different temperatures—you may want lots of ice or you may want room-temperature drinks.

When it's time to eat, you may not feel hungry but instead only tired or queasy. You might have to remind yourself to eat instead of relying on feeling hungry to prompt you to eat. By being aware of your mealtimes, staying on a schedule and eating regular small meals, you can keep the worst of the nausea away.

MEDICAL ALERT

If you have severe nausea or vomiting, or you can't keep fluids down for more than 12 hours, call your doctor for instructions or go to the emergency room for treatment.

GO FOR GINGER: NATURAL NAUSEA REMEDY

For thousands of years, ginger has been part of traditional medicine practices all over the world. Many cultures have used various forms of ginger for its natural anti-nausea properties. Recently, scientific studies have shown evidence that ginger is effective for relieving the nausea caused by chemotherapy. Ginger doesn't relieve nausea for everyone, but it's safe, inexpensive and worth giving it a try.

♥ **HELPFUL HINT**

Not everyone finds ginger helpful for nausea, and some even find that it makes nausea worse. Experiment and do what's best for you.

You can find many forms of ginger for sale, such as natural ginger root, crystalized ginger, hard or chewy candies and ginger tea. If your regular grocery store doesn't stock ginger candy, try a natural food grocery, the cancer center gift shop or online. Look for one hundred percent natural and organic ginger products, if possible. Natural ginger root can be used to make homemade ginger tea. See recipe below.

Ginger Products Resources

- Buddha Tea
- Gem Gem (candies)
- The Ginger People (candies and chews)
- Harney & Sons Ginger Licorice Tea
- Traditional Medicinals Tea
- Yogi Tea

Recipe for Homemade Ginger Tea

- 1-inch peeled ginger root, sliced into thin rounds
- Four cups water
- Juice of one lime or ½ lemon
- Agave nectar or honey

Bring the water to a boil and add ginger slices. Simmer the ginger slices in the water for 10–20 minutes, longer for stronger tea. Remove and discard the ginger. Add the citrus juice and sweetener to taste. Enjoy hot or cold. Serves four.

MEET MARY JANE: MEDICAL MARIJUANA FOR NAUSEA

Marijuana is the common name for the two varieties of the cannabis plant that are used recreationally and medicinally. Many states have legalized marijuana for medical use, and as of this writing, 11 states and the District of Columbia have legalized both medical and recreational marijuana. As more people gain legal access to cannabis, there is more interest in using marijuana to relieve nausea and other symptoms caused by chemotherapy.

Current research shows that marijuana reduces nausea and vomiting in chemotherapy patients. Marijuana plant products have different effects and side effects, depending on if they are smoked, vaporized or eaten. Preliminary studies have shown that inhaled marijuana is more effective at reducing nausea than the ingested form. However, marijuana (like all herbs) can contain trace amounts of microorganisms such as fungi. Chemotherapy patients who smoke marijuana when their immune system is low have a risk of serious infection from these germs. Patients who choose to use marijuana during chemotherapy treatment should be aware of these risks and perhaps avoid smoking as the route of ingestion.

⬦ DEFINITION: CANNABINOIDS

Cannabinoids are the active chemicals of the cannabis plant. Cannabidiol (CBD) is a cannabinoid that has anti-nausea, anti-inflammatory and pain-relief properties, and can be derived from the hemp plant. CBD is not psychoactive. A different cannabinoid, tetrahydrocannabinol (THC), causes marijuana's euphoria and psychoactive effects—its "high."

Synthetic cannabinoid medications are an alternative to marijuana. These medications, dronabinol and nabilone, are legal by prescription in all US states. Dronabinol and nabilone can be prescribed in addition to the usual anti-nausea medications for chemo patients with severe symptoms.

Cannabidiol (CBD) oil is another cannabis product that is available nearly everywhere. CBD oil is derived either from hemp or marijuana and may or may not contain any tetrahydrocannabinol (THC), the psychoactive component of marijuana. There is limited but growing evidence that CBD oil has anti-inflammatory properties and is helpful for pain, fatigue and insomnia. Similar to marijuana products, CBD oil is not FDA-approved or regulated. Thus, there is no way to guarantee the quality, purity or even the content of a particular product. Nevertheless, many people are finding CBD helpful for a variety of symptoms. As more research on CBD oil and marijuana safety and effectiveness becomes available, the cancer community will certainly benefit.

> **⚠ MEDICAL ALERT**
>
> At this time, national cancer treatment guidelines do not recommend whole-plant marijuana or CBD products for the treatment of cancer or chemotherapy-induced nausea.

GET TO THE POINT: ACUPUNCTURE FOR NAUSEA

Are you tired of ginger candy yet? Or maybe your nausea just won't quit . . . If your nausea is bad, consider acupuncture. Just as acupuncture has been shown to be effective in treating peripheral neuropathy, many studies of acupuncture show that it also reduces nausea due to chemotherapy. Several organizations, including the National Cancer Institute and the National Comprehensive Cancer Network, recommend acupuncture in their treatment guidelines.

> ### ◆ DEFINITION: ACUPUNCTURE
>
> Acupuncture is a traditional Asian medicine practice in which very thin needles are inserted into the skin and deeper tissues at specific points. According to traditional theory, this treatment stimulates energy along lines called "meridians," which leads to improvement in symptoms.

There is still debate about *how* acupuncture improves nausea—there is not a clear scientific explanation for why it works. But the scientific evidence is mounting that it does work. Research continues, and in the meantime, many patients report benefiting from this safe option to decrease nausea.

> ### ⚠ MEDICAL ALERT
>
> Make sure that if you visit an acupuncturist that they are a licensed acupuncture practitioner. In the US, licensing is controlled by each state.

Acupuncture Resources:

- National Center for Complementary and Integrative Health at https://nccih.nih.gov/health/acupuncture http://www.mayoclinic.org/tests-procedures/acupuncture/basics/definition/PRC-20020778
- National Certification Commission for Acupuncture and Oriental Medicine at https://www.nccaom.org/

AVOID STRONG SMELLS: ODORS CAUSE NAUSEA

Seriously, the topic of nausea never seems to end. During chemotherapy, just the smell of food cooking may make you nauseous. To minimize your nausea prior to meals, stay out of the kitchen whenever possible while meals are being cooked. If you must do the food preparation, fix a cold meal instead (think sandwiches, hummus, cheese and crackers) because cold food tends to have less odor and triggers less nausea. You will find more details about food and food preparation in "Chapter 4: Nutrition," later in the book.

> ♥ **HELPFUL HINT**
>
> To reduce mealtime nausea, try eating cold foods, since the aroma of cold food is usually not as strong.

It's not just food odors that can nausea—home and body product odors can as well. Switch to unscented soaps and lotions, or those with softer, naturally-derived scents such as lavender and chamomile. Avoid strongly scented cleaners and household products, such as air fresheners, if you find that these bother you. Usually this sensitivity to smell goes away after chemo is over, so you should be able to enjoy your favorite products and perfumes again in the future.

TRAFFIC JAM: CONSTIPATION

Constipation is common during chemotherapy. This is caused by a direct toxic effect of the chemo drugs on your intestines, as well as by not eating enough fiber or drinking enough water because you feel nauseous. To make things worse, some anti-nausea medications, such as ondansetron, can cause constipation. During chemotherapy you can get caught in a cycle of nausea and constipation, with a bloated belly, afraid of painfully passing a hard stool.

🏷️ DEFINITION: CONSTIPATION

Hard stools or infrequent bowel movements and difficulty passing stool, often accompanied by abdominal cramps.

Prevent constipation by drinking plenty of water in small amounts throughout the day. Eat foods high in soluble fiber, such as fruits, vegetables, beans, lentils and oatmeal. If you find it hard to eat these foods, take a daily psyllium fiber supplement, such as Metamucil or FiberCon.

⚠️ MEDICAL ALERT

Do not use enemas as they can injure the rectum and cause bleeding and infection.

Talk to your oncologist or chemotherapy nurse to find out if your particular chemo regimen tends to cause constipation. If so, consider starting an over-the-counter medication such as polyethylene glycol (Miralax) powder daily, or every other day, as a preventive measure. Polyethylene glycol is not a stimulant laxative and it works by drawing more water into the intestine to prevent constipation. For most people, it is safe to take polyethylene glycol daily to prevent constipation.

Constipation Medications, Over-the-Counter

Too late for prevention? If you are already constipated, keep up your fluids and fiber and add a daily medication for constipation. Try one from the sample regimen below.

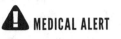 **MEDICAL ALERT**

Do not take magnesium products if you have kidney problems. Ask your doctor before starting any new medication or supplement.

- Polyethylene glycol (Miralax) powder, one scoop daily in eight ounces liquid
- Sennosides (Senekot-S), one tablet twice daily for three days
- Bisacodyl (Dulcolax), 5mg, one or two tablets at bedtime for three days

If no bowel movement by day three after chemo, take one dose of:

- magnesium citrate, 5–10 ounces, or
- magnesium hydroxide (Milk of Magnesia), 30ml (two tablespoons)

Fiber Resources

- High-Fiber Food List at **https://www.webmd.com/ cholesterol-management/features/fiber-groceries**
- Soluble Fiber Primer at **https://www.todaysdietitian.com/ newarchives/120913p16.shtml**

⚠ MEDICAL ALERT

Call your doctor for severe abdominal pain, dizziness, fever (oral temperature of 100.4F or more), rectal bleeding or continued constipation even after treatment.

ON THE GO: DIARRHEA

As often as constipation, chemo can also cause diarrhea. The direct toxic effects of chemotherapy on the lining of the intestinal tract cause poor absorption of fluid and nutrients. This, as well as not eating well during chemo, leads to diarrhea.

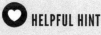 **DEFINITION: DIARRHEA**

Frequent, watery or loose stools, sometimes associated with stomach cramping.

It sounds crazy, but just as fiber helps prevent constipation, eating more soluble fiber can prevent diarrhea. This is because soluble fiber absorbs water and helps regulate bowel function. Foods that are high in soluble fiber include vegetables, fruits, beans, lentils, flax seeds and oatmeal. Try eating small amounts of these high-fiber foods several times a day and drinking plenty of water.

> **♥ HELPFUL HINT**
>
> For raw skin around the anal area due to diarrhea, try witch hazel moistened pads followed by zinc oxide cream or paste (diaper cream). Apply after each bowel movement.

If you have persistent diarrhea after a chemo cycle, with more than five–six watery stools per day, try the over-the-counter treatments below. Even if you are able to drink fluids, you may not be able to drink *enough* to keep up with the fluid loss of the diarrhea. This can cause you to become dehydrated or low on electrolytes, such as potassium. Once you have several watery stools in a row, consider taking one of the over-the counter medications listed below.

Diarrhea Medications, Over-the-Counter

- Bismuth subsalicylate (Pepto Bismol), two tablets, then repeat in four hours. Do not exceed the maximum recommended dose per 24-hour period.
- Loperamide (Imodium), 2mg tablets. Take two tablets, then repeat in four hours. Do not exceed the maximum recommended dose.

If these diarrhea medications aren't working and you are still having frequent watery stools, call your oncologist.

Fiber Resources

- High-Fiber Food List at **https://www.webmd.com/cholesterol-management/features/fiber-groceries**
- Soluble Fiber Primer at **https://www.todaysdietitian.com/newarchives/120913p16.shtml**

⚠ MEDICAL ALERT

Call your doctor for severe abdominal pain, dizziness, fever (oral temperature of 100.4F or more), rectal bleeding or continued diarrhea. Ask your doctor before starting any new medication or supplement.

HYPER AND HUNGRY: SIDE EFFECTS OF STEROIDS

Have you found yourself eating an entire box of doughnuts in one sitting? Or wondering why you suddenly have neck acne? It might be the 'roids! Corticosteroids are strong anti-inflammatory medications that are frequently given with chemotherapy to reduce nausea or to treat allergic reactions. Common corticosteroids include dexamethasone, methylprednisolone, prednisone, prednisolone and hydrocortisone. Steroids are great at preventing nausea; however, they have common side effects such as increased hunger and insomnia. Most people do not get all the side effects listed below, but it is very common to get a few. On my chemo days, I found myself up until 2 AM on the phone with my brother who lives in an earlier time zone. It took me a few cycles of chemo to realize that it was the steroids that were keeping me up that first night.

Review the list below so that you know what to look for and can report any side effects to your oncologist.

Side Effects of Corticosteroids

- hyperactivity
- insomnia
- irritability and moodiness
- high blood sugar (especially for people with diabetes)
- acne
- increased appetite
- weight gain
- swelling and fluid retention

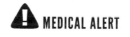 **MEDICAL ALERT**

Tell your doctor if you experience severe symptoms from this list of steroid side effects. You may need to have your medications adjusted.

YOUR PERSONAL SAUNA: HOT FLASHES AND CHEMOTHERAPY-INDUCED MENOPAUSE

If you have found yourself awake at 4 AM, overcome by waves of heat and sweat droplets prickling your skin . . . Welcome to "chemopause!" Chemotherapy frequently causes hot flashes in both women and men. This happens because chemo interrupts the body's sex hormones and creates a state similar to female menopause, sarcastically nicknamed chemopause by the cancer community. For young women, chemotherapy often shuts down menstrual cycles for the duration of treatment. This low-estrogen state lasts throughout treatment and may resolve when chemo is finished. However, for some women, this chemotherapy-induced menopause becomes permanent: the ovaries never resume estrogen production and women become post-menopausal. For men, hot flashes should resolve after chemotherapy is finished.

> ### ⬛ DEFINITION: HOT FLASHES
>
> Episodes of heat and flushing of the skin, usually starting on the face and neck and progressing to sweats. Hot flashes occur around the time of female menopause in women, or in this case, for both men and women during chemotherapy.

If hot flashes are severe, they can interrupt sleep and daily activities. Sleep is important, so don't ignore these symptoms and try to power through it! If hot flashes are disrupting your sleep or making it hard to function, ask your doctor about getting treatment. Many prescription medications have been shown to reduce hot flashes. However, some medicines cannot be taken if you have had breast cancer or other hormone-sensitive cancers, so use this list to discuss medication options with your doctor.

Medications for Hot Flashes

- Citalopram, 10mg once daily
- Clonidine, 0.1mg twice daily
- Duloxetine, 60mg once daily (cannot be taken with tamoxifen)
- Estradiol (estrogen), dosage varies, cannot be taken in breast or gynecologic cancers
- Gabapentin, 300mg three times daily
- Paroxetine, 10mg once daily (cannot be taken with tamoxifen)
- Venlafaxine ER, 75–150mg once daily

♥ **HELPFUL HINT**

If you can't take duloxetine for your hot flashes because you are on tamoxifen, try venlafaxine instead. These two medicines are similar, but venlafaxine is safe to take with tamoxifen.

If you want to avoid medications, consider this: acupuncture, aerobic exercise and hypnosis all reduce hot flashes, according to current research. These non-pharmacological approaches are safe, and exercise has many other health benefits. The only downside to acupuncture and hypnosis may be cost, since medical insurance usually does not cover these treatments.

⚠ MEDICAL ALERT

If you have had breast or gynecologic cancer, do not take estrogen. The latest research shows that it is safe to eat whole soy foods such as tofu, edamame and soy drinks. Ask your doctor before starting any new medication or supplement.

Research on natural supplements for hot flashes is not as clear, but there is some evidence that the following supplements lessen hot flashes: melatonin, 5–30mg at bedtime; omega-3 fatty acids (DHA/ALA), 2000mg daily; and soy isoflavones. It might surprise you that many popular supplements used for hot flashes have been shown to be *ineffective* when tested in formal research studies. The supplements that *do not* work for hot flashes include black cohosh, dong quai, evening primrose, ginseng, red clover and vitamin E.

COUNTING SHEEP: INSOMNIA

If you find yourself lying in bed, eyes wide and staring at the ceiling, then join the club! Trouble sleeping is common during chemotherapy. Even when you are exhausted, you might have trouble settling your mind to drift off to sleep. Worry, pain, night sweats or nausea are some of the many things that might keep you awake. Occasional loss of sleep is not usually a problem. But if you find yourself awake night after night, worn out during the day or unable to think due to fatigue, then your sleep problems are more than a nuisance . . . you have insomnia and you can do something about it.

> ### ⬥ DEFINITION: MELATONIN
>
> A natural brain hormone involved in regulating sleep. Melatonin is produced by the pineal gland in response to darkness and peaks overnight. In the United States, melatonin is available as a supplement without a prescription.

The first basic steps to improve sleep are known in the medical field as "sleep hygiene." These steps have been well-publicized in the health news and may seem self-evident: we need to avoid caffeine, noise, light and over-stimulation. Now we also know that we need to limit our media device use before bed so that the light from these devices doesn't interfere with our brain's production of melatonin, a natural sleep hormone. Some other sleep-inducing tactics are not as well-known, such as bathing earlier in the evening to allow the body to cool down before getting into bed. According to studies, the drop in body temperature appears to induce sleep.

These sleep hygiene measures have been shown to be helpful, but the biggest barrier for us is actually doing them! Review the list below as a reminder of how to set yourself up for a successful night of sleep.

Basic Steps to Improve Sleep

- Treat any pain, nausea and other physical symptoms as best as you can.
- Keep your bedroom dark, quiet and cool enough to be comfortable (69 degrees Fahrenheit has been shown to be ideal).
- Avoid drinks with caffeine after midday, or at all if you are very sensitive to caffeine.
- Begin your bedtime routine early enough to allow eight hours in bed for sleep.
- Bathe at night and allow 30–60 minutes between bathing and bedtime for your body to cool down. Studies have shown that this temperature cycling induces sleep.
- Put down your back-lit electronic devices (smart phone, tablet, lighted e-readers, television) at least 30 minutes before bedtime.
- Do not use the television to put you to sleep—stop watching TV 30 minutes before bedtime.
- Try these supplements at bedtime: calcium citrate, 200–500 mg; magnesium, 100–250 mg; or melatonin, 3–30 mg.
- Drink a cup of chamomile tea 30 minutes before bedtime.
- Do a relaxation practice such as guided breathing, prayer, meditation or mindfulness.

> ⚠ **MEDICAL ALERT**
>
> Headache and vivid dreams are possible side effects of melatonin. Start with a low dose and increase slowly. Ask your doctor before starting a new medication or supplement.

While we can't always read or listen to soothing music in the evenings, try to make your bedtime routine as calming as possible. Some people find that an aromatherapy diffuser with calming scents, such as lavender or bergamot, is helpful. If you read at bedtime, choose a print book or a non-lit e-reader. Electronic screens interfere with sleep because light from the device enters your brain through your eyes and interferes with the brain's normal nighttime production of melatonin, a brain hormone that is important for sleep.

Talk to your doctor if you still have trouble sleeping after using the techniques above. You may need a referral to a therapist for cognitive behavioral therapy for insomnia (CBTI), or a prescription medication for sleep, depression or anxiety. The next section discusses medications and severe insomnia in more detail.

> ❤ **HELPFUL HINT**
>
> If you are bothered by thinking about your "to-do list" as soon as you lie down, write the list on paper and put it on your nightstand before going to bed.

Sleep Resources

- https://www.cancer.gov/about-cancer/treatment/side-effects/sleep-disorders-pdq#section/_3
- https://www.drweil.com/health-wellness/body-mind-spirit/stress-anxiety/breathing-three-exercises/
- https://www.oncolink.org/support/side-effects/other-side-effects/insomnia/tips-for-managing-sleep-problems-insomnia
- https://www.sleepfoundation.org/

SLEEP RX: SEVERE INSOMNIA

Still awake? If you have tried the techniques for better sleep and you still have insomnia, it may be time to see your doctor to discuss the problem. Most importantly, insomnia can be a symptom of anxiety and depression, both of which are common when people are dealing with cancer and other serious illnesses. Talk to either your oncologist or your primary care doctor about both your problems sleeping and how you're feeling in general. While it's normal to have feelings of stress, anxiety, sadness and a whole assortment of other emotions, it's important to try to sort out if clinical depression or anxiety is actually the root cause of the insomnia. You can read more about anxiety and depression later in the book.

To treat insomnia, your doctor may refer you to a therapist, either for cognitive behavioral therapy (CBT) for insomnia or for help with handling the tough emotions of undergoing chemo. CBT for insomnia has been shown to be just as effective as prescription sleep medication. The biggest barrier to CBT is a lack of therapists licensed to perform this specific type of therapy and the time that it takes to do the therapy. If you can find a psychotherapist in your area who is experienced in CPT for insomnia, I strongly recommend this treatment to improve sleep and overall well-being.

Prescription sleep medication is another important option for insomnia treatment when the sleep hygiene techniques are not helping you get rest. This is especially true for the insomnia due to chemotherapy, which is usually temporary but can be severe. There is no shame in taking a medication when it is needed—sleep is necessary and chemo is stressful stuff!

Different sleep medications work in different ways, so make sure to discuss your symptoms with your doctor. This will ensure that you get the correct medication, tailored to your symptoms. Do you have trouble falling asleep? Do you wake up in the early morning? Are you anxious?

Are hot flashes waking you up? Be sure to ask about possible side effects such as sleepwalking, morning grogginess and the risk of addiction.

Common Prescription Sleep Medications

- doxepin (Sinelor)
- eszopiclone (Lunesta)
- hydroxyzine (Vistaril)
- lorazepam (Ativan)
- ramelteon (Rozerem)
- trazodone
- triazolam (Halcion)
- zaleplon (Sonata)
- zolpidem (Ambien, Intermezzo)

⚠ **MEDICAL ALERT**

If you have a history of alcohol or substance misuse disorder, several sleep medications are not recommended due to their addictive potential. Discuss risk of addiction with your doctor before starting any sleep medication.

Take any medication according to your doctor's recommendations and use the sleep hygiene techniques in the previous section to make your bedtime routine calming and regular. With some attention to what happens overnight, you can make your days a whole lot better.

RUNNING ON EMPTY: ENERGY

As you go through cycles of chemo, your energy level will cycle as well, and you may find that fatigue is a problem for you. Usually fatigue is the worst during the first few days after each treatment and your energy then returns after a week or so. You will learn your pattern after a few rounds of chemo, and this will help you plan work and social activities. Many people find that a good day with lots of energy is often followed by a low energy day. Remember to use these energy boosting techniques to help you feel your best.

Energy Boosters

- Eat regular meals and snacks, with protein at each meal. Read more details about eating during chemo in "Chapter 3: Nutrition."
- Drink enough water, approximately one ounce for every two pounds of body weight every day (unless water is specifically restricted by your doctor due to a kidney or heart condition).
- Exercise—yes, exercise! Studies show that people who exercise throughout chemotherapy have more energy.
- Get enough sleep, at least seven–eight hours per night.
- Take naps when you feel tired, limited to 30–60 minutes long. Longer naps can make you feel groggy because you enter a deeper phase of sleep. Don't nap if you can't sleep at night.
- Breathe. When we feel stress, we often hold our breath unconsciously. This can lead to muscle tension, pain and fatigue. When you are tired, pause to take ten deep breaths.

> ♥ **HELPFUL HINT**
>
> Use a journal, paper chart or digital app to track treatments, symptoms, medications and side effects. This can show you patterns and keep track of questions for the doctor.

As the months of chemotherapy go by, it is normal to feel more and more fatigued. Know your limits. Pay attention to what is happening in your body today and what you need to feel energized. Have you eaten enough? Do you need a nap? Fresh air? A hug? Go get what you need. Allow yourself to slow down if your energy is low. Regroup and reassess. Do not place demands on yourself. When you are having a good day, go for it! There is no right way to have cancer, no chemo rulebook. Instead, meet yourself wherever you are each day.

Symptom Tracking Resources

- Carezone app at **https://carezone.com/home**
- Eva app at **http://eva-app.co/**
- Living With app (from Pfizer) at
  https://www.thisislivingwithcancer.com/living-with-app
- Navigating Care website at
  https://www.navigatingcare.com/patient/
- NCCS Pocket Cancer Care Guide at
  https://www.canceradvocacy.org/resources/pocket-care-guide/

WORK THAT BODY: EXERCISE

It may surprise you to learn that exercise improves your energy level during and after chemo. Studies show that people who exercise while they are undergoing chemotherapy treatments are less fatigued than those who do not exercise. Exercise improves flexibility, strength and balance. It also strengthens the immune system and balances stress hormones. Exercise is healthy for you, even during chemotherapy, so make a plan to get moving.

If you can, try exercising several times per week, but don't feel pressure to overdo it. This is not the time for a no-pain-no-gain attitude. Chemotherapy causes loss of muscle mass, resulting in weakness and a higher risk of injuries. If you have anemia (low red blood cell count), you may get dizzy and winded easily. During the middle part of my chemo treatment, I was very anemic, and my exercise consisted of a slow walk a few mornings per week before the heat of the day became intolerable. If you are not in the habit of exercising, remember to start easy and increase your workouts slowly. Try a low-impact workout such as an elliptical trainer, stationary bike, tai chi or swimming for 15–30 minutes every other day to start. If you had a vigorous workout routine prior to chemotherapy, reduce the intensity of your training and monitor how you feel.

♥ HELPFUL HINT

If you are capable of only minimal physical activity, try breathing exercises such as those found at https://www.doyogawithme.com/yoga_breathing or insighttimer.com.

Exercise Resources

- ChoosePT at **https://www.choosept.com/Resources/Detail/ top-10-ways-exercise-helps-during-cancer-treatment**
- NCCN exercise resources at **https://www.nccn.org/patients/ resources/life_with_cancer/exercise.aspx**
- Self Magazine at **https://www.self.com/ gallery/9-low-impact-workout-moves-you-can-do-at-home**
- Women's Health Magazine at **https://www.womenshealthmag. com/fitness/a19930648/no-equipment-workout/**

⚠️ MEDICAL ALERT

Public gyms are often contaminated with bacteria such as methicillin-resistant Staphylococcus aureus (MRSA). MRSA infection can be fatal for people with a weak immune system, such as during chemotherapy. Do not use the gym when your immune system is weak.

PHYSICAL THERAPY: GET HELP WITH EXERCISE

Do you sometimes feel like you have woken up in someone else's body? No, you haven't been abducted by aliens—you're just noticing what surgery, radiation and chemotherapy are doing to your body. You may have pain, scars or tightness. There may be a part of your body that is damaged or absent due to treatment. Exercise may seem impossible right now, but it's not. Exercise is more important than ever before, but you might need some guidance to find the right way to go about it.

Get to know your new body by working with a physical therapist or rehabilitation doctor (physiatrist). Your family doctor or oncologist can refer you to a physical therapist or to a physiatrist in your area. Physical therapy will teach you exercises that you can do at home given your current physical capabilities. You can regain strength and learn to work with any new characteristics of your body. If surgery is planned as the next part of treatment, doing physical therapy before surgery will strengthen you and help you recover faster.

DEFINITION: PHYSIATRIST

A physiatrist is a doctor who specializes in physical medicine and rehabilitation. This specialty focuses on restoring or improving function and quality of life for patients facing physical impairments or injuries.

Physical Therapy Resources

- American Cancer Society at https://www.cancer.org/treatment/survivorship-during-and-after-treatment/staying-active/physical-activity-and-the-cancer-patient.html
- Cancer Exercise Training Institute at https://thecancerspecialist.com/free-essentials-of-cancer-exercise/

- ChoosePT at **https://www.choosept.com/Resources/Detail/ top-10-ways-exercise-helps-during-cancer-treatment**
- HEP2GO Exercise Builder site at **https://www.hep2go.com/index_b.php?**
- National Center on Health, Physical Activity and Disability at **https://www.nchpad.org/Videos/ PLwMObYmlSHaN0Pbu2xXymDUePlsTCsn7n**
- Verywell Health at **https://www.verywellhealth.com/ physical-therapy-exercises-4013311**

CHEMO BRAIN: COGNITIVE DYSFUNCTION

Not only will your body be tired at times during chemo, but your brain will be too. Many people feel like their brain doesn't work properly during chemotherapy, and they report symptoms such as memory problems, difficulty learning new things, trouble concentrating, confusion or trouble staying organized. Chemotherapy patients have nicknamed this phenomenon of brain dysfunction "chemo brain." Chemo brain isn't an actual clinical diagnosis, but the brain dysfunction and memory symptoms associated with chemotherapy are real. These chemo-associated brain problems are starting to be better studied and described. Chemo brain symptoms appear to be caused by a combination of the direct effects of chemotherapy drugs on the brain, plus other factors such as stress, fatigue, menopause, insomnia, anxiety and pain.

Not everyone gets chemo brain—some people seem to come through chemotherapy with no brain dysfunction whatsoever. Generally, the symptoms of brain dysfunction will improve after chemo is over, but for some people the symptoms persist after treatment is finished. Despite this, a large study recently confirmed what earlier studies showed: that people diagnosed with cancer are at a *lower* risk of decline in brain function, memory problems and dementia. The reasons for this are not clear, but research is ongoing.

⚠ **MEDICAL ALERT**

Call 911 or go to the emergency room if you have any of the following neurologic symptoms: weakness or numbness on one side of your face or body, slurred speech or sudden loss of vision. These symptoms can indicate a possible stroke.

If you have any problems with thinking and memory, tell your oncologist. It's possible that you may have a different medical problem that is causing the symptoms, such as low thyroid function, a vitamin deficiency or anemia. Thyroid problems and nutrient deficiencies are treatable problems, but they can mimic chemo brain symptoms. Your doctor may run specific blood tests or other exams to check for these and other problems. Depression and insomnia can also cause difficulty with memory and concentration, and they are also treatable.

In addition to seeing your doctor about symptoms of chemo brain, you can take basic steps to take good care of your brain. Although it may seem simplistic and obvious, it's very important to follow these basic health practices:

- Get enough sleep (at least seven–eight hours per night, more if you feel that you need it)
- Drink enough water (1 oz per kg body weight per day/1 oz per two pounds body weight per day)
- Avoid drinking alcohol or using recreational drugs
- Eat enough (see "Chapter 3: Nutrition")
- Use relaxation practices if you are in a state of activated threat response (see chapter 1)

NO TROPHY FOR SIDE EFFECTS

The cancer-fighting effect of chemotherapy is not related to whether the treatment gives you unpleasant side effects. If you are breezing through treatment and feeling good, then be thankful! Don't worry that this means that your chemo isn't working. There is no connection between how well the chemo works and how severe the side effects of the chemo are.

On the other hand, if you are struggling with constipation, or you can't eat because of nausea or mouth sores, don't despair. Take a moment to gather your strength, then step up your efforts to treat these problems. If you've already adjusted your preventive medications and you're still suffering, ask for help: call your oncologist's office to speak to the chemo nurse, or make an appointment with your oncologist. You will not get a trophy at the finish line for having endured the worst side effects!

Don't feel like a failure if your side effects are bad—you didn't bring this on yourself. Similarly, if your side effects are minimal, let go of any guilt that might come from comparing your situation to someone else's situation whose suffering might seem greater than yours. There is no right or wrong way to go through chemo. Allow things to be as they are and let go of expectations—yours or anyone else's.

VISUALIZE THE WAY FORWARD

Are you midway through your chemo triathlon now, sweating and cramping, aching and blistering? Is the hardest hill still ahead? Or has chemo been easier than you thought, and you're only beginning to tire?

Now is the time to hold steady, to maintain your effort and to keep the goal in sight. When chemotherapy is completed, you will be able to recuperate, regroup and enter the next phase of recovery. Take a moment now and use this visualization exercise to notice how your chemo is helping and healing you and to appreciate how strong you are.

Visualize the Way Forward

Imagine the chemo destroying the cancer cells and your immune cells working to protect you. Feel the energy from the food that you eat strengthening your body. Imagine the oxygen from each breath rushing into your cells and refreshing you. Feel proud of your body for all that it is doing for you. Feel proud of being present and brave.

CHAPTER 3

PREVENTING INFECTION

KNOW YOUR NADIR: WHEN YOUR IMMUNE SYSTEM IS LOW

Most chemotherapy suppresses the body's immune system. After each chemotherapy treatment, your immune cells will decrease in number, and the period when the immune cells are lowest is called the nadir. During the nadir you are the most vulnerable to infections.

✎ DEFINITION: NADIR

The period of time after each chemotherapy treatment when your immune system is suppressed to its lowest point and you are most prone to infection.

Some chemotherapy regimens, such as those for leukemia and breast cancer, are very suppressive to the immune system, causing a long and severe nadir. Regimens for other types of cancer do not cause the immune cells to decrease nearly as much. Your oncologist will tell you when to expect that your immune cells will reach their nadir after each cycle of chemotherapy and how long the nadir will last.

The time when your immune system is in the nadir is when you need to take the strictest precautions to avoid infection. Note that if you are being treated while hospitalized with very aggressive chemotherapy, such as for leukemia or before a stem cell transplant, you may spend a long time in a nadir. In this case, your immune system will be low for weeks to months at a time, and you must follow precautions to prevent infection during the entire treatment period. In the sections that follow, you will learn several ways to prevent and monitor for infection.

MONITORING FOR FEVER

At some point during chemo, you are likely to have a fever. While the fever could be signaling a common cold that your six-year-old brought home from school, fever can also be a sign of a more serious illness. An oral temperature of 100.4F or higher can be a sign of dangerous infection such as pneumonia or sepsis (blood poisoning). When you are undergoing chemotherapy, you must be observant and take symptoms seriously— even if you were likely to brush them off in your life before cancer.

> ### ⬛ DEFINITION: SEPSIS
>
> A serious, full-body reaction to infection that affects many organs. It can cause low blood pressure, kidney injury, fluid imbalances, liver injury and confusion. Some people with sepsis require treatment in the intensive care unit. People who have immune system suppression from chemo are prone to sepsis, but sepsis is treatable when detected and treated.

Throughout chemotherapy, get in the habit of checking your temperature anytime you feel warm, sweaty, chilled, achy or just more tired than usual. Have an oral digital thermometer at home that is only for you (i.e., not shared with other family members). Make sure that you have not had anything to eat or drink for 15 minutes prior to taking your temperature, since that can change the temperature of your mouth and cause an inaccurate reading. If you do register a temperature of 100.4F or higher, don't panic. You may be just overheated from extra clothing or blankets. If that might be the case, take off some layers and recheck your temperature in 15 minutes. If your temperature is still 100.4F or more, however, call your oncologist immediately. Even if it's after hours, the on-call doctor will call you back with instructions.

You may want to keep a treatment journal or use an app to keep track of your chemo treatments and any symptoms, including your temperature. However, try not to worry and obsess about every detail. Remember that this is new territory for you, and it's not your job to figure everything out! Observe your body so that you can report what you notice to your doctor.

> **⚠ MEDICAL ALERT**
>
> If you have an oral temperature of 100.4F or higher, call your oncologist even if it is after office hours. Fever can be a sign of serious infection.

Symptom Tracking Resources

- Carezone app at **https://carezone.com/home**
- Eva app at **http://eva-app.co/**
- Living With app (from Pfizer) at **https://www.thisislivingwithcancer.com/living-with-app**
- Navigating Care website at **https://www.navigatingcare.com/patient/**
- NCCS Pocket Cancer Care Guide **https://www.canceradvocacy.org/resources/pocket-care-guide/**

A BOOSTER SHOT: COLONY-STIMULATING FACTOR INJECTIONS

Many types of chemotherapy can cause severe immune suppression (a very low nadir). If your chemotherapy regimen causes this, your oncologist will likely order an injection of a medication called colony-stimulating factor, which will stimulate your immune system. You will receive this injection on the day after each chemo treatment. These shots prevent a very low nadir by stimulating the bone marrow to produce more immune cells. This decreases your risk of getting a serious infection and helps prevent delays in treatment due to low blood counts. The names of the colony-stimulating factors are filgrastim (Neupogen, Granix, Zarxio) and pegfilgrastim (Neulasta).

Be aware that colony-stimulating factor injections usually cause significant side effects, the worst of which are bone and muscle pain. Take acetaminophen (Tylenol) or ibuprofen (Advil, Motrin) to prevent and minimize the discomfort caused by immune-boosting shots.

Colony-Stimulating Factor Side Effects:

- bone pain
- muscle and body aches
- headache
- fatigue
- low-grade fever (oral temperature 99–100.3 F)

💙 **HELPFUL HINT**

Some people find that taking the allergy medication loratadine 10mg on the day of chemo and daily for the next three days prevents the body aches that often arise after receiving a colony-stimulating factor injection.

LIMIT CONTACT: AVOIDING INFECTION BY STAYING IN

Many infections, such as colds, influenza and intestinal infections, are passed from person to person by direct contact. My boys were in elementary school when I was diagnosed with cancer and began my chemotherapy. At that age, kids bring home enough germs on a daily basis to infect an army! Because of the intensity of my chemo, the severity of my nadir (the time when the immune system is low) and my boys' high infectious risk, I had to implement a strict no-contact rule at my house during my nadir. This meant no kissing, no touching hands and hugging only with my self-invented No-contact Nadir Hug method. At bedtime, after they had showered and were ready for tuck in, I would wrap the kids head-to-toe in a blanket, like a taco, and hug them through the blanket.

Luckily, nadir is short and limited—I didn't have to resort to hugging kid tacos that often! But, nevertheless, it's important to avoid infection by limiting physical contact during your nadir. You can limit the risk of catching an infection during your nadir by not shaking hands or kissing and by limiting your contact with people. This means that it is best to avoid crowded places and events, such as church, schools and stores. During your nadir is a time when you need to delegate tasks such as shopping to your loved ones who want to help you. Also avoid social events with people who might be ill or having visitors to your home who are sick.

> ❤ **HELPFUL HINT**
>
> Be brave about asking if anyone is sick before they come visit you—and tell them not to come! Your visitor might not remember that a simple cold can be very dangerous for you!

If you work in healthcare, education or childcare, you may not be able to work at all during your nadir, since your workplace is a source of germs that can cause infection. Even if your job does not involve a high level of contact with people, ask your doctor about when you should avoid work. See chapter 1 for information about taking disability leave from work and for resources to protect your job.

OUT AND ABOUT: AVOIDING INFECTION IN PUBLIC

No matter how cautious you are, there will be times when you will be in your nadir (and at high risk for infection) and yet need to be around people or go out in public. This is not ideal but will often be unavoidable. When you find yourself in these situations, use these methods to prevent picking up germs from public places:

- Greet people with a "fist bump" or "elbow bump" instead of a handshake or hug.
- Blow a kiss hello instead of giving a kiss on the cheek.
- Use alcohol-based hand sanitizer frequently and carry it with you in your car, purse and briefcase. Use sanitizer after every skin contact, after using the restroom and before meals.
- Have alcohol-based hand sanitizer available on your desk at work and at home near the front door.
- Train yourself to keep your hands off your face and use a tissue for scratching or wiping, since most germs are carried to the openings on the face (eyes, nose, mouth) by the hands and fingers.

> **⚠ MEDICAL ALERT**
>
> Ask your doctor if and when you should wear a medical face mask in public places.

- Wash your hands frequently: after using the restroom, before eating or preparing food and immediately upon arriving home or getting back to the office.
- Use the back of your hand or a paper towel when touching faucets in public restrooms.
- Open public restroom doors with a paper towel or part of your clothing after you've washed your hands.

POSTPONE THE DENTIST

Unless it is an emergency, postpone any routine dental work and cleanings until chemotherapy is finished and your immune system is back to normal. Dental work, including routine cleaning, loosens mouth bacteria and causes tiny areas of trauma to the gums. Bacteria enter your bloodstream through these tiny abrasions. While not dangerous under normal circumstances, when your immune system is suppressed by chemotherapy, even such mild damage can cause a life-threatening infection.

Take good care of your mouth and teeth during chemo by treating your mouth gently. Brush your teeth carefully twice daily with a soft toothbrush and use a sensitivity toothpaste if your gums are sore. Avoid mouthwashes that contain alcohol or other disinfectants because they can irritate the gums. Instead, use a moisturizing mouth rinse, such as Biotene, and avoid using a tongue scraper, since this will traumatize your tongue. Do not floss during your nadir because flossing releases bacteria into your bloodstream and can cause serious infection.

> ♥ **HELPFUL HINT**
>
> Schedule a routine dental cleaning before chemotherapy begins, since you should not have cleanings during chemotherapy.

STAY CONNECTED: AVOID LONELINESS DURING YOUR NADIR

If you're stuck at home because of a low immune system during your nadir, you're probably going to feel isolated. Even when your immune system is strong, you may be too tired or nauseous to go out and socialize. Sometimes even talking on the phone takes too much energy.

Counteract loneliness by remembering to reach out to those around you. I found that being at home with my family was very comforting. My younger son, an optimist by nature and nine years old at the time, had this to say about my summer of chemo: "Having chemo is 60 percent bad because you're sick . . . but it's 40 percent good because you can stay home and play board games with me." You too might discover a new activity or hobby by spending more time at home with loved ones—I learned to play Othello, although I still don't win!

Allow visitors in small numbers, as long they are healthy. Texting takes less energy than talking, so text with family and friends if you are too tired to talk. Consider connecting with people face-to-face through video conferencing, such as Zoom or Skype, or use FaceTime. Seeing other people, if only through a computer screen, will do wonders for your spirits. If you like social media, you can connect that way: post an update to your media page or chat online in a cancer support group. Facebook has many general cancer support groups and groups for caregivers, as well as disease-specific groups. Recently, these groups have become better monitored and focused on creating a safe place for support and sharing information. Twitter and Instagram also have cancer-related support groups. Several health-specific platforms, such as Navigating Cancer (**https://www.navigatingcancer.com/**) and CaringBridge (**https://www.caringbridge.org/**), offer customizable websites where you or your caregiver can upload information to keep everyone updated about your treatment. Using technology and social media as part of your connection strategy avoids always having to update everyone individually. You can keep your loved ones informed without wearing yourself out.

AVOID FOOD POISONING: FORBIDDEN FOODS DURING CHEMO

Eating well is one of the ways you can keep yourself healthy during chemotherapy. Good food is good medicine. But if food becomes contaminated with bacteria or other germs, it can cause food-borne illness, often called "food poisoning." When your immune system is weak from chemotherapy, food poisoning can be extremely dangerous. Symptoms of food poisoning are stomach pain, nausea, vomiting, diarrhea and fever. In severe cases, food poisoning can cause dehydration and sepsis, a severe response to bacterial infection that affects the entire body. Certain foods are high risk for bacterial contamination, and to avoid food poisoning, you should avoid them for the entire chemotherapy treatment period.

> ⚠ **MEDICAL ALERT**
>
> During chemo, leftovers are allowed for the next day only. Eat them or throw them out after 24 hours.

Forbidden Foods

- No raw seafood, such as sushi, raw shellfish or oysters.
- No rare meat. All meat should be cooked well-done.
- No fresh cheeses, such as fresh mozzarella, queso fresco (fresh Mexican cheese) or feta cheese. (These cheeses usually come packed in water.)
- No unpasteurized dairy products, such as raw cheese or milk.
- No unpasteurized juices, either bottled or freshly squeezed from a juice bar. Bacteria multiply quickly on juicing equipment and without the heat of pasteurization.
- No kombucha, kimchi or other fermented and unpasteurized foods.
- No buffet or picnic food.

- No leftovers more than 24 hours old, even from home-cooked food.
- No raw foods at restaurants, such as salads, berries and uncooked salsas. (See how to disinfect raw vegetables and fruits at home in the section that follows.)
- No raw or partially cooked eggs. This means no Caesar salad dressing made with raw eggs, no eggs with runny yolks, no uncooked meringue and, unfortunately, no raw cookie dough!

⚠ **MEDICAL ALERT**

If you have an oral temperature of 100.4F or higher, vomiting or diarrhea that lasts more than 24 hours or severe stomach pain, call your oncologist even if it is after office hours.

RINSING IS NOT ENOUGH: DISINFECT RAW FRUITS AND VEGGIES

Raw fruits and vegetables are an important part of your diet. They contain fiber, vitamins, live enzymes, antioxidants and many other healthy components. However, fruits and vegetables can carry harmful bacteria and parasites on their surfaces, and they must be disinfected if you want to eat them raw. During some chemotherapy regimens, such as for leukemia, your doctor may tell you not to eat raw vegetables at all. If you are allowed to eat raw veggies and fruits, which is the case for most people during chemo, be sure to wash and disinfect them.

Disinfecting is cheap and simple with a home-made vinegar spray. Use the following recipes for a disinfecting solution made from household white vinegar to disinfect fruits and vegetables before eating them raw. This spray can also be used to deodorize cutting boards after cutting onions and garlic if you find that the odor is strong and causes nausea.

Vinegar Disinfecting Spray for Vegetables and Fruits

Combine white vinegar and filtered water in a spray bottle in a ratio of 1:3 and shake to combine.

1/2 cup white vinegar

1 1/2 cups filtered water

Spray onto vegetables or fruits, coating all surfaces, and let sit for two minutes

Rinse well, drain and prepare as usual

Spray disinfect all vegetables and fruits that you plan to eat raw, such as grapes, apples and tomatoes. Even vegetables that you peel, such as carrots and cucumbers, should be washed, disinfected and then peeled. For fruits that you slice, such as melons, thoroughly wash the outside with running water, then disinfect the outside of the fruit with the vinegar spray, rinse again, then slice.

Many veggies and fruits, such as berries, have wrinkles and grooves that are hard to reach by spraying. Leafy greens, herbs and berries must be disinfected by immersing in a vinegar soak. This includes all salad greens! If you want to eat these raw, wash first, then place in a vinegar soak, then rinse again to remove the vinegar.

> ♥ **HELPFUL HINT**
>
> If the fruits and vegetables will be completely cooked, such as by roasting, steaming or sautéing, you can skip the disinfecting but be sure to wash them thoroughly.

Vinegar Disinfecting Soak for Leafy Greens and Berries

2 cups white vinegar
6 cups filtered water
Combine white vinegar and filtered water in a large mixing bowl or basin
Soak the greens/berries for ten minutes
Rinse thoroughly with running water
Drain and dry, then prepare as usual

IT'S NOT JUST RESTAURANTS: CLEAN KITCHEN TECHNIQUE

We like to blame food poisoning on eating out, but foodborne illness is often from contamination at home. In addition to disinfecting all raw fruits and vegetables, good practices will prevent your kitchen from becoming a source of bacterial contamination.

Clean Kitchen Technique

- Wash all cutting boards, knives and countertops with soap and hot water immediately after preparing poultry and meats.
- Consider switching to wood cutting boards instead of plastic, since wood is naturally anti-bacterial.
- Throw away dish sponges frequently, and change kitchen towels every day.
- Clean your countertops with a disinfecting spray, preferably one with bleach.

> ♥ HELPFUL HINT
>
> Heat your damp kitchen sponges in the microwave daily for two minutes on high to sterilize them. Throw them out after one week.

Remember, you have lots to do! If these cleaning tips are too much work, use paper towels and other disposables for the duration of chemo and don't feel guilty about it!

SAVE THE JUICING FOR LATER

Making homemade juice from fresh fruits and vegetables has become very popular, and people drink homemade juice to increase their intake of vitamins, antioxidants and natural live enzymes. However, juicing is risky during chemotherapy due to trace bacterial contamination on the fruits, vegetables and equipment. When your immune system is low, your body can't fight off the germs that it normally would. If you want to juice, you will need to carefully disinfect all vegetables and fruits that you put into the juicer. In addition, all parts of the juicer will need to be taken apart, washed and run through the dishwasher on a sanitize cycle to sterilize it, every time you juice. Every. Single. Time.

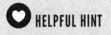

HELPFUL HINT

Make a homemade vinegar and water disinfecting spray to disinfect your raw fruits and vegetables. Use one part white vinegar to three parts filtered water.

I decided not to juice during chemo—it was too time-consuming and too risky! It is safest to postpone juicing until after chemotherapy when your immune system is back to normal. You can get the same benefits as juicing from eating raw fruits and vegetables in their whole form, with the added benefit of their natural fiber. And remember, always wash and disinfect all vegetables and fruits that you eat raw.

MEDICAL ALERT

The juicer needs to be washed and sanitized (sterilized) every time you use it, and all fruits and vegetables need to be washed and disinfected before juicing.

EATING OUT: WHEN IS RESTAURANT FOOD SAFE?

> **♥ HELPFUL HINT**
>
> Bring plastic utensils with you to restaurants to reduce the risk of infection and avoid the metallic taste from metal utensils.

Who wants a break from cooking and cleaning up the kitchen? You do! But there is no guarantee that the restaurant food was prepared properly to prevent contamination. Foodborne illness, such as salmonella or cryptosporidium, is common and frequently associated with restaurants. No one is as careful as you are. For this reason, unfortunately, it's best not to eat at restaurants during your nadir (when your immune cells are at their lowest point in your chemotherapy cycle).

When you are not in your nadir and your immune system is strong, eating out is safe as long as you stick to cooked foods only. Remember, at all times during chemo you should avoid rare meat, undercooked eggs, fresh cheese, raw milk and raw seafood.

> **⚠ MEDICAL ALERT**
>
> Only eat out in restaurants when your white blood cell count (immune system) is normal, not during your nadir.

FURRY FRIENDS: PREVENTING INFECTION FROM PETS

When chemo is making you sick, having your dog or cat curled up next to you can be a great comfort. But pets also carry germs, so now is the time to outsource the more unpleasant tasks such as litter box duty! Look at these tips to enjoy your pet safely and avoid getting an infection.

Tips for Pet Safety to Prevent Infection

- Wash your hands thoroughly with soap and water after petting or playing with your pet.
- Make sure that your pet is up-to-date on all vaccinations.
- Do not clean the cat litter box.
- Do not clean bird or animal cages.
- Do not pick up dog feces.
- Do not allow your pet to lick your face.
- Do not sleep with your pet.

Pets are experts at giving us that unconditional love, so take a few steps to stay safe and you can keep your pets snuggled close.

HAVE PATIENCE

Do not despair; your nadir will not last forever. For most chemotherapy regimens, the period of lowest immune function lasts for about one week after each round of chemo. Your doctor may order blood tests between treatments to determine when your immune cells are back to normal. Knowing your blood counts will tell you when your nadir starts and ends, which tells you when you must follow the strictest measures to avoid infection.

The cancer world is a world of paradox: despite being on high alert, try not to worry too much. Focus your efforts on infection control during your nadir, then allow yourself to live a bit more normally when your blood counts are normal. Focus on doing things that you control, such as disinfecting your vegetables, cleaning your hands well and exercising at home instead of the gym. This will conserve your energy and your state of mind. Try the visualization exercise below to boost your brave factor and gather your infection-fighting energy.

Gather Infection-Fighting Energy
Visualize your immune cells bouncing back after each round of chemo. Feel the cells circulating in your body, defending you against germs. If a thought or fear about infection appears, notice it and let it go, like a passing cloud. Remember that all the actions you take, and the habits you build to protect yourself from infection, are creating a safe wall of protection around you. You are strong and ready to continue your chemo.

CHAPTER 4

NUTRITION

t's time to feed the machine. This is a challenge, remember? Food is your fuel to heal your wounds, take your journey or fight your battle. Eating during chemotherapy is different than eating before you had cancer. You can't just reach for whatever food is available, and you may not be able to rely on your hunger pangs to tell you that it's time to eat. Your favorite foods may no longer appeal to you and you won't be able to go all day without eating, if that was your previous routine. Eating needs to become your new full-time job.

Prepare your mind to fuel your body because you will have to overcome obstacles to eating. You will need to eat even when you have no appetite, when you are nauseated and when it hurts to swallow. To keep your body strong, you need to eat food that is full of energy and nutrients. Ideally, you would eat this way all the time, but because of the numerous side effects that chemo can cause, it's often difficult to eat anything during chemo—never mind eating healthfully! To help you manage your diet in the healthiest and most comfortable way possible, this chapter reviews what to eat and why, with resources on nutrition during chemo for those who want more details.

WHAT TO EAT: CHEMO NUTRITION IN A NUTSHELL

There are entire books written on nutrition and cancer. Nutrition for prevention of cancer, nutrition during treatment and nutrition during recovery. Right now, you need the basics. You need core concepts that you can implement to keep yourself fed, strong and feeling good. If you have the energy and time, there are resources listed at the end of this section that will give you more details, but for now, start with these core guidelines.

- Eat whatever you can manage. If you are struggling to eat due to mouth pain, nausea or poor appetite, then remember this: Eat whatever is comfortable, whatever you can keep down and whatever appeals to you. Just eat something!
- Eat something with protein at every meal. This will keep your energy up, reduce nausea and help prevent muscle loss.
- Eat a small meal or snack every few hours. Popular choices are crackers, watermelon and popsicles. Don't let an empty stomach make nausea or fatigue worse.
- Eat as many fruits and vegetables as possible, making sure they are cooked or disinfected thoroughly.
- Choose whole grains over processed grains to increase fiber, vitamins and minerals. This includes brown rice, whole wheat, corn tortillas and old-fashioned oats.
- Limit sweets and desserts, especially sugary drinks like soda, since these foods have little or no nutritional value.
- Avoid spicy foods, hot foods and foods with strong smells if these foods make you nauseous, or if spicy foods hurt your mouth.
- Drink eight–ten glasses of water and other non-caffeinated drinks per day, unless your doctor has told you to limit fluid intake.

Resources for Nutrition During Chemo

- *Anticancer: A New Way of Life.* Servan-Schreiber MD PhD, David. Reprint edition. Penguin Books, 2017.
- *The Cancer-Fighting Kitchen, Second Edition: Nourishing, Big-Flavor Recipes for Cancer Treatment and Recovery.* Katz, Rebecca, and Mat Edelson. Revised ed. edition. Berkeley: Ten Speed Press, 2017.
- Chemocare website, nutrition section at http://chemocare.com/chemotherapy/health-wellness/managing-nutrition-during-cancer-and-treatment.aspx
- *What to Eat During Cancer Treatment.* Besser, Jeanne, and Barbara Grant. Second edition. American Cancer Society, 2019

PACK IN THE PROTEIN

Your muscles, bones and tissues are made of protein. Eating enough protein is essential for energy, maintaining your body's tissues and proper
organ function. Under stress, such as illness and chemotherapy, your
protein requirement increases. Eating some protein at every meal, or as
a snack, will give you more energy throughout the day, prevent nausea
and help prevent loss of muscle mass. Try snacking on these protein-rich
foods throughout the day to meet your body's needs.

High-Protein Foods

- Meat. Can't argue with the protein content of meat.
- Cheese sticks or slices. High in protein, calcium and fat. If your
  mouth is sore, try cottage, ricotta or cream cheese.
- Hummus (garbanzo bean puree), or any other bean puree. Use as
  a dip for vegetables, or spread on
  crackers, toast or pita bread. High
  in protein and fiber.
- Peanut butter, almond butter, or
  sunflower seed butter.
- Nuts, all kinds. Roasted, not raw
  because of infection risk.
- Canned tuna or canned chicken
  breast. Mix with mayonnaise or
  olive oil for a quick salad.
- Cooked beans, any kind. Use
  canned, or dry beans cooked from scratch.
- Yogurt, regular or Greek style.
- Eggs, hard-boiled or other style of fully cooked eggs.
- Whole milk. If you are losing weight, drink a glass of whole milk
  daily for the protein, fat, calcium and calories.

> ♥ **HELPFUL HINT**
>
> Estimate how many grams
> of protein you need to eat
> per day by dividing your
> weight in pounds in half.
> Example: 180lb divided
> by two = 90g of protein
> needed per day.

- Soy "milk," unsweetened. High in protein and lower in sugar than dairy milk.

If you find that you can't eat enough food to keep up your protein intake, high-protein meal supplements, such as protein bars and shakes, are also a good option. Popular brands of protein drinks include Ensure, Boost, Vega, Orgain, Svelte and Atkins. Big box stores also make similar and affordable "house brand" versions of these bars and shakes.

♥ HELPFUL HINT

Protein drinks also come in a "clear" variety that is dairy-free and soy-free. These clear versions are compatible with the "clear liquid diet" that your doctor may prescribe if you are vomiting or having stomach pains.

Protein Smoothie

Protein powder of choice
(whey, soy, plant-based)
Milk of choice (dairy, soy,
almond, oat, rice)
½ cup of fruit, frozen or
fresh (disinfected)

> ### ⚠ MEDICAL ALERT
>
> Beware of high sugar content in pre-packaged shakes and bars. Read the label and choose carefully if you need to watch your sugar intake.

Optional sweetener to taste: honey, agave syrup, Stevia
1 tablespoon of add-ins: wheat germ, ground flax seeds, raw rolled oats, hemp seeds

Blend ingredients in a blender until smooth and enjoy.
May be kept in the refrigerator for 24 hours.
Remember to disinfect raw fruit and sanitize the blender after each use.

SNEAK IN A SNACK

As you read previously in the sections about nausea, you need to avoid an empty stomach. Snacks are not only important for preventing nausea, but snacks will provide you with calories and nutrients when you find it impossible to eat a full meal. Plan on stocking up on snacks and eating them throughout the day, every two to three hours. This will provide you with calories and nutrients, as well as prevent nausea.

Healthy snacks are best, such as whole grains, fruits, cheese sticks or other protein-packed foods. However, when you are nauseous and your appetite is poor, don't stress out about what you're eating. Remember that it's better to eat *something* rather than *nothing*!

❤ HELPFUL HINT

Don't wait until you are hungry to eat a snack. You may never feel hungry because chemotherapy interferes with the nerve signaling that controls taste, smell and hunger.

EAT YOUR VEGGIES AND GRAINS

I'm gonna say it: kale. It took me three months and five recipe failures before my husband and kids would eat it. I thought the family favorite would be kale cooked with bacon, but it turns out that they like it Cuban style the best—sautéed with olive oil and lots of garlic. I guess we have my husband's Cuban heritage to thank for that!

Eating more vegetables and fruits is a challenge for most of us, but it's worth it. Now more than ever, during chemo you need vegetables and fruits for fiber, prebiotics, minerals and vitamins and even for water. Aim for five servings per day, with one serving being about ½ cup cooked or one cup fresh.

During chemo your taste buds are distorted, so kale may not be the vegetable of choice to go for. Instead, choose gentler veggies such as carrots and green beans. Acidic vegetables and fruits, such as tomatoes and citrus, may burn your mouth if you have mucositis, so eat these with caution.

> ❤ **HELPFUL HINT**
>
> If you don't have the time or energy for washing, disinfecting and cooking fresh vegetables and fruits, remember that you can buy them canned, frozen or packaged.

For grains, choose whole grains over processed grain products whenever possible. Whole grains provide fiber, which prevents constipation and diarrhea, as well as iron, magnesium and protein. This means eating whole wheat bread instead of white, corn tortillas instead of white flour and brown rice instead of white. In my family, switching to brown rice from white took even longer than learning to like kale. We live in a border town near Mexico where making typical Spanish rice using brown rice is unheard of. But I did it—I now make Spanish rice using Basmati brown rice, and my husband says anything that he's willing to eat, anyone can eat!

SLAY YOUR SWEET TOOTH: REDUCING SUGAR

We all like comfort food. Near the end of chemo, I recall bingeing on some vegan chocolate-chip cookies that a friend made for me. And I did it while binge-watching an old TV show—that's how far gone my brain was!

However, while chocolate and good television are great for the soul, a high-cookie, high-sugar diet is not great for the chemo patient. There is evidence that eating excess sugar and processed starches can increase inflammation and insulin levels, both of which can lead to harmful effects such as weight gain, diabetes, chronic pain and cardiovascular disease. I made a great effort to cut my sugar intake as much as possible at the start of chemo, and despite my hereditary sweet tooth, I still try to maintain a low-sugar diet.

If you want to begin reducing the sugar in your diet, start by taking an inventory of what you eat over a few days. Do you eat dessert frequently? If so, perhaps you can cut down by half. Do you sweeten your coffee? Try leaving out the sugar. It takes about a week for your palate to get used to unsweetened coffee.

Speaking of coffee, drinks are a common source of sugar that is easily eliminated. Instead of sugar-sweetened drinks such as soda, sports drinks and sweet tea, try drinking water or unsweetened tea. Even natural fruit juice contains lots of sugar! Yes, it's natural sugar but it's still sugar. You get greater benefits from eating the whole fruit, such as fiber and live enzymes, and drinking a glass of water, than from drinking fruit juice.

The next step for sugar reduction is to find hidden sources of sugar. For most of us, a large source of hidden sugar is the added sugars found in processed foods. Added sugars are sugars that do not occur naturally in a food but are added to the food when processed. To discover this sugar source, you will have to read food labels. Added sugars include ingredients such as sucrose, maltose, high-fructose corn syrup, rice syrup and honey.

In an ideal world, we would never eat packaged or processed foods and all our food would be home cooked. Of course, in an ideal world none of us would be having chemotherapy either! In real life we eat processed or packaged foods for convenience, such as commercially prepared breads or cereals, energy bars and frozen dinners. These items are frequently necessary, but even so, it is possible to find healthy options. When you buy prepared foods, check the labels and choose foods low in added sugars. Look for products labeled as whole grain as well. You will notice that whole grain foods (e.g., corn tortillas) usually have less sugar than "white" or processed grain foods (e.g., flour tortillas). Once you make the habit of checking the labels for sugar content and reaching for whole grains instead of white or processed grains, you will dramatically decrease your sugar intake.

TAKE A MULTIVITAMIN

Even if you are doing a good job of eating a variety of foods and maintaining your weight, a daily multivitamin is recommended for most people during cancer treatment. A basic multivitamin plus minerals will do. Nothing fancy or expensive is needed. If you are drinking meal replacements such as Ensure or Boost, these are vitamin-fortified, and you do not need to take an additional multivitamin.

Some people have deficiencies of iron, vitamin B12, folate and vitamin D. Ask your doctor if you need to be tested for these deficiencies or should be taking the following supplements during chemotherapy:

- iron (ferrous gluconate or ferrous sulfate)
- calcium (calcium citrate is preferred)
- vitamin D-3
- Omega-3 fish oil (DHA/ALA)
- B vitamins

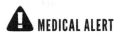 **MEDICAL ALERT**

Ask your doctor before you start taking any new vitamin or supplement.

HOLD THE ANTIOXIDANTS: NO SUPPLEMENTS DURING CHEMO

Do you have well-meaning friends who urged you to take cancer-fighting supplements? Have you fallen down the internet rabbit hole of cancer miracle-cures? Preliminary research shows that many natural compounds such as green tea, alpha-lipoic acid, resveratrol and many others have anti-cancer properties. Many of these compounds are available as oral supplements and are being tested in clinical studies to see if they can prevent or treat cancer, either alone or in combination with chemotherapy and other conventional cancer treatments.

> ⚠ **MEDICAL ALERT**
>
> Do not take antioxidant supplements such as green tea, curcumin, alpha-lipoic acid, resveratrol or even vitamin C while you are undergoing chemotherapy. These may make chemotherapy less effective.

So far, the research results for most supplements have been mixed depending on the dose, the type of cancer cell, the delivery method and many other variables. Many supplements have been tested only in the laboratory in cell culture or in animals—not in humans. While some studies do show that several supplements have beneficial cancer-fighting effects, in other studies many supplements seem to *protect the cancer cells* from the action of the chemotherapy. For this reason, until more research is performed, you should not take most supplements while you are still receiving chemotherapy. The risk is too great that the supplements may interfere with the cancer-fighting effectiveness of your chemotherapy. Remember, always ask your oncologist before starting a vitamin or supplement.

FROZEN AND DELICIOUS: GETTING YOUR VEGGIES WITHOUT DISINFECTING

Too tired to disinfect your fruits and veggies? It's a drag having to spray and soak raw fruits and veggies with disinfecting spray. Sometimes you need a fast, simple solution to getting fruits and vegetables in your diet. Here's a list of prepared vegetables and fruits that are safe to eat right out of the package.

Safe and Easy Fruits and Veggies

- Applesauce. Add cinnamon or nuts to make it interesting.
- Mixed fruit cups packed in water.
- Tomato juice or other vegetable juice, preferably a low salt version. Tomato is high in lycopene, a cancer-fighting natural compound, and low in sugar.

> **⚠ MEDICAL ALERT**
>
> Watch for food recalls. There have been outbreaks of *Listeria* and *E. coli* bacteria, which can cause severe infection, even in healthy people. Look up food recalls at https://www.foodsafety.gov

- Frozen berries. Cook on the stovetop until hot, then cool and mix with yogurt, or add to a protein smoothie. High in vitamins, antioxidants and fiber.
- Canned mixed vegetables. Add to canned tuna or canned chicken breast for a variation on tuna/chicken salad.
- Frozen vegetables and greens. Easy to cook in the microwave or sauté with olive oil.

WHEN EVEN WATER TASTES BAD: STAYING HYDRATED

♥ HELPFUL HINT

Avoid drinking excessive sports drinks and soda since these are high in sugar. Sports drinks are helpful if you have diarrhea because they replace electrolytes such as sodium and potassium.

During chemo, sometimes even the taste of water can make you nauseated. But you need to drink lots of fluids to flush the chemotherapy and the dying cancer cells out of your system. You should be drinking enough fluids each day so that you urinate several times per day and your urine is a light yellow color. If your urine is dark or you haven't urinated in more than eight hours, this means that you are not drinking enough fluids. If you're a person who likes to keep track of numbers, a good estimate of the number of ounces of fluid to drink per day is half of your weight in pounds (for example, 140 pounds/2= 70 ounces per day). Try these tips to make water taste better and get enough fluids each day.

Tips for Tasty Water

- Drink water purified by reverse osmosis
- Drink sparkling water, plain or flavored
- Add a squeeze of lemon or lime
- Add slices of cucumber or disinfected mint leaves
- Add sugar-free flavor drops
- Add a splash of sports drink or juice

⚠ MEDICAL ALERT

If you have heart or kidney disease, you may have restrictions on the amount of daily fluid that is safe for you to drink. In this case, ask your doctor.

In addition to water, you can also stay hydrated by drinking herbal tea (iced or hot), natural juices and sports drinks. Black tea and coffee are also fine in moderation, but stay away from alcohol. Alcohol is dehydrating, and it's a neurotoxin (it damages nerve cells).

TRUST THE NUTRITION BASICS

You have so much to do right now. Work, bills, kids. Appointments, tests, chemo. The importance of eating can get lost in the chaos or drowned out by nausea. So remember the basics: Eat small, frequent snacks and don't wait to feel hungry. Eat foods that are high in protein. Stay hydrated by drinking lots of water. Choose whole grains and limit your sugar intake where you can. Above all, the most important thing is to eat whatever food your body can tolerate right now. Remember that your body is an expert at digesting and absorbing all the food you give it. Use this exercise to tune in to your body's expert power.

Power Food

Take a moment to think about what you ate today. That wasn't just food, it was power. You are powering your cells with the food that you eat. Crunchy, soft, chewy, salty or spicy—it's all coursing through you now and becoming part of you.

Trust your body—your body knows how to rebuild you with the fuel that you give it: new parts, new cells and new defenses.

Feel proud of yourself for powering up your cells today. With every bite you are closer to being healthy.

CHAPTER 5

APPEARANCE MATTERS

Up to now, we've spent a lot of time discussing and managing your internal workings: your immune system, your digestive system and your energy level. But external aspects are also important. Your appearance is important. Why? Because it's your interface with the world. It's the first impression others have of you, and it's a barrier of protection for you. Your appearance is also a form of self-expression, a way for you to communicate to others. It is something that you can choose and control, to some extent, even during chemotherapy.

Your appearance may have changed drastically, or it might change soon if you are just starting your chemo. If this happens, it can be terrifying. A slightly deranged analogy that came to my mind at the start of my chemo was that having chemo was like being pregnant. It's a time when your body is completely taken over and reshaped by another force. But instead of having a baby at the end of the pregnancy, it was I who would be reborn at the end of chemo. A bit nutty—I know—but somehow this metaphor helped me to put up with the physical derangements that I was experiencing!

So how can you manage this hostile takeover of your body and your self-image by chemo? Finding your mindset is helpful. Go back and work on that if you skipped those sections. Managing your appearance is another way. This chapter discusses ways to handle the challenges that you will face in your body, from hair loss to weight changes to dry skin, and how to take back your image and make it your own again.

ATTENTION CONEHEADS: DEALING WITH BEING BALD

Here we are again, back to hair loss. Previously, I discussed how to prevent it, how to postpone it and how to make it less painful. Now let's talk about how to handle it. Once you're bald, how do you think you will feel about that? Some men are prepared to look like Mr. Clean, and some women embrace the "bald looks better with earrings" look. Will you feel energized and free once you are free of hair? Some people are heartbroken, having lost what they feel is their best feature. Do you think you will dread seeing yourself in the mirror? Whatever you feel about being bald, *that's how you feel*. And that's just fine.

Once hair loss is firmly underway, it is common to experience your hair falling out in clumps. At this stage, many people decide to shave their heads. I couldn't stand the patchy look, so my husband helped me to buzz off the remaining clumps of hair in the backyard with his beard trimmer.

Moving on to practical matters, will you cover your bald head? Some people choose to go bald in public if the weather permits. You also might be pleasantly surprised at the shape of your scalp and opt to decorate it with henna or other temporary tattoos. Allow yourself some fun with the bald option.

Do you want to wear a wig? What about a head scarf or hat? There are many hats that are specially designed for people who are bald due to chemo and other medical conditions. These hats are made extra-deep to cover the tops of the ears and the bare area at the back of the head. Some hats even come with hair sewn in around the back and side brims. If you think that you want to wear a full wig, consider having a custom wig made from your own hair. This is possible if you have at least ten inches of current hair length. Wigs will be covered by insurance with a doctor's prescription for a "cranial prosthesis" and a diagnosis code for chemotherapy-related hair loss.

When planning how to handle being bald, think about the season: will it be warm or cool by the time your hair falls completely out? Will you be commuting to work or spending most of your time at home? Consider what will make you feel most like yourself and least vulnerable. Start with these basic tips for taking care of your bald scalp and for planning how to protect your head when needed.

Scalp Care and Coverage

- If you plan to buy a wig, get a prescription from your oncologist for a "cranial prosthesis" and order in advance, since custom wigs can take up to eight weeks.
- Buy a few scarves or caps before your hair starts to fall out, so that you are prepared. Most oncology practices also have a selection of donated scarves and caps that are free to patients.
- When your hair starts falling out in clumps, consider shaving off the rest. Try the first pass with clippers and then remove the stubble with a razor.
- Wear a brimmed hat, such as a beach or fishing hat, whenever you are outside. This protects both your scalp and your neck.
- Use sunscreen with SPF 30 or higher on your scalp and neck, even if you don't plan on being outside. Wear sunscreen even on cloudy days because chemo makes your skin burn more easily.

Headwear, Scalp and Wig Resources

- Caring and Comfort at **https://www.caringandcomfort.com/**
- Compassionate Creations at
  https://www.compassionatecreationswigdesign.com/
- Cure Diva at **https://www.curediva.com/**
- Hats for You at **https://www.hatsforyou.net/**

- Headcovers Unlimited at
  https://www.headcovers.com/scarves/head-scarves/
- Henna Tattoos on Live Better with Cancer website at
  https://cancer.livebetterwith.com/blogs/cancer/cancer-henna-crowns
- Look Good Feel Better (Australia) at https://lgfb.org.au/
- Look Good Feel Better (Canada) at https://lgfb.ca/en/
- Look Good Feel Better for Men at
  http://lookgoodfeelbetter.org/programs/men/
- Look Good Feel Better (United Kingdom) at
  https://www.lookgoodfeelbetter.co.uk/
- Look Good Feel Better (United States) at
  http://lookgoodfeelbetter.org/ 1-800-395-LOOK (5665)
- Tender Loving Care from American Cancer Society at
  https://www.tlcdirect.org/

TAKE CARE OF YOUR SKIN

Skin can become dry and take on a gray color during chemotherapy. Some chemo medicines deposit in the skin and cause color change. Anemia (low red blood cell count) also changes the appearance of the skin and, depending on your natural skin tone, your skin can look ashy, yellow or pale.

Good skin care is important in order to avoid cracks in the skin that can allow infection to set in. Begin by bathing with warm but not hot water. If your skin is dry, you may want to use cleanser only on your oily or sweaty parts, such as underarms, genitals, feet and skin folds. Use a gentle cleanser, preferably unscented, and moisturize your skin with a non-irritating skin cream as soon as you finish bathing. Avoid products with heavy perfumes, as perfumes can cause nausea and be irritating. Common brands that make unscented products include Alba Botanical, Aveeno, Burt's Bees, CeraVe, Dove, Garnier SkinActive and Kiss My Face.

> **⚠ MEDICAL ALERT**
>
> If you see any cut, crack or sore on your skin that is getting red, swollen or has drainage, tell your oncologist. You may have a skin infection and need antibiotics.

Remember to care for your lips and eyes as well. Frequently apply lip balms with natural oils such as coconut, avocado, jojoba and beeswax. Your tear ducts and the oil glands of the eyelids may not produce as much lubrication during chemo, and this can cause dry eyes. For this, use moisturizing eye drops such as Refresh or Systane. It sounds backwards, but watery eyes can be a sign of dry eyes, so apply lubricating eye drops frequently throughout the day and you may have less tearing.

Losing your fingernails and toenails is also a problem with some chemo regimens. Using cooling booties and mittens during chemotherapy infusion, if available, might help avoid this. Keep your nails trimmed short and inspect them daily for cracks or signs of infection. Some patients have had good results with applying tea tree oil to their nails to avoid nail loss. There hasn't been any research to support the use of tea tree oil, but it's safe and inexpensive—thus worth a try to many people.

Some of us grew up sunbathing, but this is strictly off-limits during chemo. Many chemotherapy drugs increase sun sensitivity, so you will find that it's easier to get sunburned. This is true even if you have dark skin and don't usually get burned when out in the sun. During chemo, everyone needs to take measures to protect themselves from sunburn.

If you can, avoid sun exposure from 11 AM–3 PM, and do not use tanning beds. Use sunscreen with SPF 30 or higher on all exposed skin, and wear sun-protective clothing with a UPF rating of 50 or higher. Remember to wear a hat with a full brim to protect your scalp and your neck. Protect your eyes with sunglasses that have a 100 percent UV rating. By taking preventive measures, you can soak up the happiness from the sun's rays and avoid the burn!

Resources for Skin Care

- Alba Botanical (for natural sunscreens, face and body care) at
  https://www.albabotanica.com/en/
- Aveeno brand (for face and body care) at
  https://www.aveeno.com/about
- Garnier SkinActive 96% Natural (for hair, face and body care) at
  https://www.garnierusa.com/
- Healthy Living smartphone app from the Environmental Working Group (for home and body products) at
  https://www.ewg.org/apps/

CHEMO CAMOUFLAGE: HOW AND WHY TO LOOK GOOD

Your last eyelash fell out yesterday. You officially have the "chemo look"—hairless and pale—which is like going out in public wearing a billboard that says, "I have cancer." Strangers may give you unwanted advice or throw you a pitying glance.

An antidote to this unwanted attention is to camouflage your chemo look. If you take steps to help yourself look healthy and more "normal," you can go out in public without feeling like a spotlight is on you. You won't have to spend your energy listening to other people's unsolicited stories about cancer or answering their questions about how you're doing. Passing for a non-chemo person allows you a mental break. This is one of the ways that looking good can help you feel better. When you take the focus off chemo and off having cancer, then you can just be you—feeling more normal and out having a regular life.

♥ **HELPFUL HINT**

Some days, you'll be too tired to fake looking normal. You'll go to the grocery store with no eyebrows, wearing sweats and a baseball cap. The world will have to deal with it.

To start recovering your fashion mojo, buy some new clothes that fit. Men, this means you too. If you have lost or gained weight, as is common during chemo, your old clothes won't fit and you can't always go out in sweatpants. Really you can't. Buy a few nice outfits that fit you well, and you'll feel better about your appearance. If you're on a tight budget, consider shopping at an upscale consignment shop, where you can find beautiful designer clothes at a fraction of the cost of new clothes. You'll feel good about looking good when you have nice clothes for appearing in public, clothes that are not baggy or tight.

If you choose to cover up your bald head, put on your wig or pick out an attractive hat or head scarf. Take advantage of the many online resources that can demonstrate ways to wear neck and head scarves.

Learn to use accessories such as jewelry, belts, scarves and headwear. Both men and women can experiment with ties, socks, shoes and hats in creative ways. I had a few mishaps doing this, since I'd never been one to wear flashy jewelry. I learned the hard way that a woman in a head scarf wearing large hoop earrings does not look awesome. She looks like a pirate.

Consider wearing makeup if you don't already. Both men and women can benefit from a good skin routine, as described previously, followed by concealers to cover blemishes or uneven skin tone. Chemo can cause skin to become pale, sallow or ashy. Even if you haven't worn makeup before, now is the time to learn to draw on your eyebrows and apply fake eyelashes. You don't have to be Instagram-ready, but taking the time to apply a little face powder, eyebrows and lipstick can make the difference between feeling like you have the face of a vampire and feeling ready to face the world. For a bolder look, try the makeup tips below:

Makeup Tips to Combat Chemo-Look

- Use foundation over your sunscreen (or foundation with sunscreen).
- Learn to draw in your eyebrows with brow liner. There are templates and online videos available for guidance if you haven't done this before!

> ♥ **HELPFUL HINT**
>
> If you have a friend who is talented at makeup and fashion, now is the time to ask for help. Or look on YouTube for a tutorial!

- Apply fake eyelashes, especially if you are going to a special event.
- Accentuate your eyes with eyeliner. Sometimes this is enough to visually compensate for a lack of eyelashes.
- Wear lipstick. Always. Be bold.
- Add color and contour to your eyes and face with eyeshadow, blush, bronzer and cheek highlights and lowlights.

Chemotherapy can be grueling, and right now you're feeling the collateral damage inside and out. Use chemo as a free pass to play with your image, and you might learn something. My brother-in-law rocked a Pitbull look during his chemo for leukemia, with a bald head and mirrored glasses. Want to buy a pink wig? Do it! Want to get a henna tattoo on your head? Do it! Sticking with a scarf or conservative wig? That's what I did! It's your decision, and when you take charge of your appearance, you'll feel better.

> **⚠ MEDICAL ALERT**
>
> Throw away old makeup when you start chemo due to the risk of bacterial contamination. Buy a new supply and treat yourself to something fun!

Chemo Appearance Resources

- Live Better with Cancer at **https://cancer.livebetterwith.com/**
- Look Good Feel Better call 1-800-395-LOOK (5665) and at **http://lookgoodfeelbetter.org/**
- For men at **http://lookgoodfeelbetter.org/programs/men/**
- Tender Loving Care at **http://www.tlcdirect.org/hair-loss-hats-scarves-turbans-caps**

A HARD LOOK IN THE MIRROR: HOW YOU FEEL ABOUT YOUR APPEARANCE

No matter how hard you try to look your best and pass for normal, there will be days when you look at yourself and see the ravages of cancer and of chemo. Who is that in the mirror? Mr. Clean? Shrek? An extra for the next zombie thriller? I have a dark sense of humor, so I could laugh at myself. If you laugh too, it's okay!

Other days, you might cry or rage or be utterly speechless. That's okay, too. You will not have the energy to put on any presentable clothing or a wig, let alone false eyelashes. You will be tired of trying to look your best, either actually tired or maybe just a fed-up kind of tired. You will stand in a check-out line or pump gas with a bald head and let people stare at you and you won't give a crap. Because even giving a crap takes energy, and right now you need that energy for you. For getting through this. For getting better.

Looking in the Mirror
Look at yourself in the mirror without a scarf or wig and without makeup. What feelings come up about your appearance? Allow the feelings to be there. It's common to feel sadness, disgust, embarrassment or a sense of loss.

If you feel these emotions, so be it. You can feel all these things and still have space for other emotions, such as hope, love and strength.

Can you feel kinship? You stand with all of us who are also bald and tired from chemo.

Can you feel wise? You have learned so much on this journey.

Can you feel proud? Your waxy skin and hairless head are symbols of what you have endured.

Can you feel brave? You've earned it.

CHAPTER 6

YOUR RESTLESS MIND

A friend of mine had completed a series of cancer treatments in the year prior to my diagnosis, and as I was about to start my own chemo, he offered this advice: "Remember, friend, it's a mind game."

This statement meant nothing to me initially, but as time passed and I began to feel more beaten down, I remembered his words. Several weeks into chemotherapy, I had suffered many setbacks: a collapsed lung, infections, low blood counts, treatment delays and the onset of neuropathy. I was more than halfway through my treatments when I found myself looking at the calendar, my eyes fixed on the last day of chemo marked with a big circle. But despite nearing this milestone, I couldn't summon joy. Instead, I flung myself face down on the bed, sobbing. The mind game had temporarily outwitted me.

Chemo is hard and complicated. Many concerns and challenges may arise, such as facing your own mortality, living with a disability or a loss of part of your body, strained family relationships and even wondering about your life purpose. The emotions that come with these issues are just as complex as the logistics of living with them. And working through these important topics requires more than just some tasty kale recipes or perky text messages with praying hands, although those help too. *To make it through chemo, you need to be aware of the mind game that chemo requires you to play.* To do this, you need to feel your emotions—all of them—and face the complex issues as they arise. The purpose of this chapter is to help you do that—I'm going to show you how to be aware of your feelings and stay mentally healthy, even when the game gets tough and the emotions are painful.

IS THERE A NEGATIVE TO POSITIVE?

Have you been told that you must stay positive? People told me to stay positive all the time, never mind that I was undergoing chemo so aggressive that I felt like I was in a horror film. I was told to "just stay positive, and you'll be fine." It was maddening. Similarly, when you aren't feeling hopeful, do you feel guilty about not trying hard enough or not praying hard enough? I felt this way at times—and most of my patients do, as well. There is even a myth that stress and negativity will make your cancer grow. This myth that stress will make your cancer grow is all over the internet, itself growing as if it were a cancer. As if you aren't already under enough stress, the pressure to avoid negativity and stress can make you feel *stressed about your stress*! These ideas are all a part of a positive-thinking trap.

Positive thinking can be tricky. Sometimes, a positive attitude is comforting and energizing. Other times, forcing yourself to think positive in the face of serious adversity can feel like a prison. It locks up the rest of your feelings and makes you feel like a fraud, smiling on the outside but raging or crying on the inside. False positivity is hurtful, exhausting and can lead to self-blame. You shouldn't suppress your natural feelings in an attempt to stay positive. When you face your feelings honestly, you will most likely realize that you have a complicated mix of emotions. This is normal because cancer is horrible, chemo is difficult and this experience is changing your life in some significant ways. It's also normal to feel both happy and sad, even about the same event or at the same time. The healthiest way through this positivity trap is to feel all your feelings, including the dark ones. Here's an exercise to help you do that.

Feel Your Feelings

How do you feel right now? Circle a few phrases on this list that click for you.

- *I can't feel anything. I'm numb.*
- *I miss my old life before cancer.*
- *I feel free to say what I really think about things now.*
- *I feel irritated by little things these days.*
- *I'm restless and want to make changes in my life.*
- *I'm hopeful that I'll have a great life when my chemo is finished.*
- *I feel jealous of other patients whose cancer is not as advanced as mine is.*
- *I feel guilty about chemo being "easy" for me, compared to other people in my support group.*
- *I'm worried that my partner won't love me anymore.*
- *I feel grateful that my cancer is responding to treatment.*
- *I'm afraid of dying.*
- *I worry about how my family will cope with my death.*

Write down some other thoughts that come to mind by completing these phrases:

- *I feel sad that:*
- *I can't stop:*
- *My biggest fear is:*
- *I wish that:*
- *I hope that:*
- *I feel better when:*
- *I'm learning that:*
- *I realize that I'm stronger than I thought when:*

Use this exercise whenever you need to make sense of your feelings or you want to find some meaning or direction from what's been happening. If you are participating in a cancer support group, this exercise can give you a starting point for topics and feelings that you might want to share with the group. Undoubtedly, you will have some shared feelings and some differences of perspective with other chemotherapy patients. Listening to experiences and opinions that are both similar to, and different from yours can be helpful as you process what going through chemo means to you. Finally, your responses to these questions may change over time as you go through treatment, or they might not. This is both normal and expected. The important step is to keep examining, keep questioning and allow yourself to feel.

EXAMINE FEAR OF DEATH

You can pretend otherwise, but once you've been diagnosed with cancer, thoughts of death are hovering in your mind, lurking in a corner. This is not surprising or abnormal—most people with cancer think about death sometimes. Facing death, or your fear of death, might be the most difficult thing that you do. Thoughts of death are there, even if you try to ignore them. Thoughts of death can squeeze out your breath and drain your hope. It's even worse if you try *not* to think about death: fears grow even bigger and thoughts of death seem even deadlier.

Thoughts of death cannot hurt you, nor do they define you. Thoughts of death will lose their power to terrify you as you sit and examine them. By allowing the thoughts to come, instead of forcing them down or avoiding them, you will likely find that over time, you will have less fear of death. You will begin to have a relationship with the thought of your dying. Try examining your thoughts of death with this exercise.

> ### *Look Death in the Face*
> *Allow the thought of death to rest in your mind. Look it in the face.*
>
> *What does death look like? Let yourself see and feel the specifics for a while.*
>
> *Allow any fear of death to come in. What are you afraid of? Are you afraid of dying soon? Of feeling pain when you die? Are you afraid of leaving your family behind?*
>
> *What are these thoughts about death telling you?*
>
> *Use these thoughts like a lens, to focus on what is important to you and on what you value for yourself and for those close to you.*

Obviously, examining your thoughts and fears about death does not make it any more or less likely that you will die from your cancer. But the more that you allow yourself to think about death and examine your fear of death, the less afraid you will be. By exploring your fear of death, you will gain a certain mastery over it and become better able to examine your mortality. And all the introspection, examination and contemplation of death can hopefully lead you to focus more clearly on your reasons for continuing through this difficult trial. You will gather some courage and perhaps some peace. When you do, you will be better able to return your attention back to your main objective: getting through your chemotherapy treatment. Although chemo is scary and miserable, chemo is your weapon, your tool and perhaps your path back to life. Regain your courage and return your attention to the task at hand. Return to braving chemo.

Resources for Coping with Fear of Death

- *A Beginner's Guide to the End: Practical Advice for Living Life and Facing Death* by Dr. BJ Miller and Shoshana Berger, Simon & Schuster, 2019
- *Being Mortal* by Atul Gawande, Picador, 2017
- *Dessert First* by J. Dana Trent, Chalice Press, 2019
- *Everything Happens for a Reason, and Other Lies I've Loved* by Kate Bowler, Random House, 2018
- *Help, Thanks, Wow* by Anne Lamott, Riverhead Books, 2012
- National Coalition for Cancer Survivorship at **https://www.canceradvocacy.org/**

EXAMINE YOUR THOUGHTS: PRACTICE MINDFULNESS

One way to observe your thoughts and emotions is to use a technique called mindfulness. Mindfulness means noticing without judgment whatever arises in the present moment, both within you and around you. In other words, being mindful means placing your full attention on what is happening and observing it in a non-judgmental way. The concept and practice of mindfulness has been around for thousands of years, and mindfulness is a key part of meditation practices such as Buddhism and yoga. However, it is not necessary to meditate or practice any particular religion in order to practice mindfulness.

Studies of mindfulness on human health show that increasing mindfulness improves sleep, blood pressure, depression, anxiety, immune function and even some biological measures associated with aging. Many studies of mindfulness have focused on cancer patients and on chemotherapy treatment and recovery. Mindfulness practice improves depression, fatigue, anxiety, sleep and quality of life during and after cancer treatment. Try this basic breathing exercise to get started practicing mindfulness.

Simple Mindful Breathing Practice

- Sit in a comfortable upright position of your choice, such as in a chair with your feet flat on the floor, or on a cushion with your legs crossed.
- Look slightly downward or close your eyes.
- Relax your eyelids, your jaw and your neck.
- Extend your spine upward by imagining a string pulling you up through the top of your head.
- Pay attention to your breath as it goes in, then out.
- Feel the sensation of the air as it enters and exits your nose.
- When your mind wanders, as it naturally will, gently bring your awareness back to the sensation of your breath.

- Notice your chest, how it expands and contracts.
- Notice if the air is warm or cool in your nostrils.
- Continue for two to three minutes, focusing your attention on your breath, and returning to the breath when your thoughts interrupt you.
- When you are ready to stop, open your eyes and take three big breaths while rubbing your palms together.

You can use this breath-focused mindfulness exercise as a starting point for your practice of mindfulness. Some people like to incorporate mindfulness as part of their morning routine. Some prefer to practice in the evening as part of relaxation before bed. The hardest part is making a daily habit of your practice. Studies of mindfulness practice show that there is benefit to even short periods of mindfulness practice. If time is limited, as it is for most of us, it is more beneficial to practice for a short time on most days, such as three to five minutes, than to try to commit to a longer practice only once a week. Most people can "steal" two minutes at some point during the day to practice a little mindful breathing. Use the websites and smartphone apps listed below to remind you and guide you in your mindfulness practice, and experiment with styles to find one that suits you best.

Smartphone Apps for Mindfulness and Meditation

- Bodhi Mind Meditations at https://www.bodhimind.me/
- Breath2Relax app, available for Apple and Android
- Calm at https://www.calm.com/
- Insight Timer at https://insighttimer.com/
- Waking Up: Guided Meditation at https://wakingup.com/

Websites for Mindfulness and Meditation

- Do Yoga With Me at https://www.doyogawithme.com/
- Glo at https://www.glo.com/
- Mindful at https://www.mindful.org/
- Melli O'Brian (Mrs. Mindfulness) at https://mrsmindfulness.com/
- National Center for Complementary and Integrative Health, Tai Chi and Qi Gong for Wellbeing at https://nccih.nih.gov/video/taichidvd-full
- Open Heart Project at https://susanpiver.com/open-heart-project/
- Sonima at https://www.sonima.com/meditation/guided-meditations-meditation/
- Qi Gong Institute at https://qigonginstitute.org/
- Tai Chi for Health Institute at https://taichiforhealthinstitute.org/
- University of California, Los Angeles Mindful Awareness Research Center at https://www.uclahealth.org/marc/body.cfm?id=22&iirf_redirect=1
- Wildmind: A Community Supported Meditation Initiative at https://www.wildmind.org/
- Yoga Journal at https://www.yogajournal.com/

Books about Mindfulness

- *The Miracle of Mindfulness* by Thich Nhat Hanh, Rider, 2008
- *When Things Fall Apart: Heart Advice for Difficult Times* by Pema Chödrön, Shambhala, 2016
- *Wherever You Go, There You Are: Mindfulness Meditation in Everyday Life* by John Kabat-Zinn, Hachette Books, 2005

MINDFULNESS ANYWHERE

You do not have to meditate, change your religion or sit cross-legged on the floor to practice mindfulness. You don't have to change your breathing or close your eyes. Being mindful just means observing and bringing your awareness to what is happening right now. At any time, you can practice mindfulness by paying attention to what you are doing.

For example, practice being mindful when you are washing the dishes or taking a shower. Notice how the water feels touching your skin, what you see and any sounds that you hear. This will have the benefit of improving your focus, making you feel less anxious and less overwhelmed.

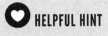

HELPFUL HINT

Practice mindfulness while waiting at medical appointments. Notice what is hanging on the wall, what sounds you hear. Feel the chair against your legs, the floor against your feet. Focus on your breathing, in and out.

MOVING MINDFULNESS

Even with the best of intentions to try a mindfulness practice, many people find it difficult to sit in formal meditation positions, such as cross-legged or with knees folded under. These positions may be painful, and it can be hard to sit still, especially for beginners. If you find it hard to be still, try moving mindfulness.

♥ **HELPFUL HINT**

Invite a friend over to practice mindfulness with you. Having a mindfulness or meditation community (even an online community) can help keep you motivated.

Go for a walk and instead of listening to music or getting lost in thought, pay attention to your surroundings and tune in to your senses. What does the air feel like against your skin? What do you smell? What is the sound of your feet as you step?

There are many forms of traditional mind-body exercise that combine mindfulness with movement, such as qi-gong, yoga and tai chi. There are numerous classes, apps, online resources and DVDs available. Some communities offer free outdoor yoga and tai chi classes, so check your local newspaper or community website for information.

TOO MUCH

Despite all the exercise, mindful walking, protein smoothies and prayers from your loved ones, on some days it's just going to be too much. Your brain is full, your tank is empty. You've got nothing left.

When this happens, it's okay to disconnect for a while and stop processing. Zone out in front of the TV. Feel sorry for yourself. Cry in the shower. Stop making an effort to be graceful in public, and don't apologize for being honest about how you feel. Don't do anything that isn't absolutely necessary. Eat off paper plates and buy thirty pairs of underwear to avoid doing the laundry.

Don't feel guilty that you aren't being strong or thinking positive or practicing mindfulness. Just be.

MORE THAN TOO MUCH: DEPRESSION

What if you can't stop crying? What if you can't think straight? What if you want to run away, run right out of your own skin? You could be depressed. Depression is common in people with cancer and can occur at any time, including after chemo is completed. Depression is sadness and hopelessness that is interfering with your ability to function, but it is treatable.

⬤ DEFINITION: DEPRESSION

Clinical depression is a medical condition defined as sadness, hopelessness and other symptoms that interfere with your ability to function and are more severe than would be expected in response to a serious illness.

Both your family doctor and your oncologist are qualified to screen and treat you for depression. Alternatively, your doctor may decide to refer you to a psychiatrist if your symptoms are severe. Your doctor will ask you about symptoms and, if you are showing signs of depression, recommend counseling and prescribe medication. Tell your doctor if you have had any of these symptoms for more than two weeks:

⚠ MEDICAL ALERT

Tell your doctor if you have thoughts of killing yourself. While thinking about or worrying about death is normal during chemo, thoughts of suicide are a sign of depression.

Symptoms of Depression

- persistent sadness
- persistent irritability (grumpiness)
- persistent hopelessness
- inability to enjoy things that usually give you pleasure

- inability to concentrate or problems with memory
- insomnia
- thoughts of suicide or a suicide plan

Other symptoms of depression include fatigue, poor appetite, weight loss and increased sleep. However, these symptoms, as well as problems with concentration and memory, can be caused by chemotherapy. You should tell your doctor about these symptoms, but they do not necessarily mean you are depressed.

MAINTAIN YOUR MENTAL HEALTH

The challenges during chemotherapy seem endless and constant—from pain and nausea to medical bills and family stress. Maybe you've screamed in anger and faced some of your fears. Maybe you've dabbled in some mindfulness and searched for a streak of personal growth in this horrendous mess. Can you keep yourself mentally healthy despite chemotherapy? Yes, you can. From a practical standpoint, attending to the following areas can help you stay on top of your mental game.

For many people, faith is a cornerstone to their wellbeing. If you are part of a religious tradition, practicing your faith can be a source of energy and comfort. Whenever you can, attend your religious services and study your holy scriptures. Prayer and meditation are healing practices, and attending religious services connects you to others who will encourage you. Even if you don't belong to a particular religious group, any spiritual practice that you keep can also provide comfort, insight and support.

Hope is also important for keeping your mental energy strong. Note that having hope, however, includes more than just hoping to be cured. Some of you may be receiving maintenance chemotherapy for advanced cancer, and in this case there will be no last day of chemo. When treatment will not bring a "cure," you must define for yourself what your hopes and goals for treatment are, such as staying healthy enough to go back to work, spending time with family or traveling. Maintaining your hope for a "good outcome," however you define it, is key to being able to live as free as possible from depression and fear. It is possible to have hope while living with an advanced disease.

Seeking the company of supportive friends and family is another way to boost your spirits. When you surround yourself with those who love you, it can help you feel happier and more hopeful. The kind words and actions of your loved ones function to fill up your emotional reserves that have become depleted. You have been working so hard to take care of yourself during your chemotherapy treatment. Allow yourself to be recharged by soaking up some good vibes from your favorite people.

Remember the power of humor to make you feel better—even gallows humor! I had a friend during my chemo treatments whose self-appointed job was to send me cards, books and jokes. Most of these were hilarious but twisted cartoons about cancer. If you have a good laugh, it will lift your spirits and release tension. You can watch a funny movie with family or friends or listen to a comedy podcast alone while lying down for a nap. If you're tired, it may be easier to listen to audio books. During chemo, sometimes things just seem ridiculous and detached from reality. You might find yourself asking, "How did I get here?" On these days, laughing seems like the only appropriate response.

Finally, don't underestimate the benefits of exercise on your mental health. Just as exercise can help your body to withstand the harsh effects of chemotherapy, exercise can help your mind. Exercise reduces anxiety, improves mental alertness and improves sleep. Even if you can't do a vigorous workout due to pain or shortness of breath, a gentle walk or stretch routine will be helpful.

Take stock periodically of your mental state. How's the mind game going? It's easy to get wrapped up in the daily logistics of appointments, work and food preparation. Make a point to ask yourself, "How am I feeling?" You can return to the previous writing exercise to do some contemplation or do some mindful breathing. Then, take whatever steps you can, literally and figuratively, to care for your own mental health.

Healing Visualization

Sit or lie in a comfortable position with your spine straight and your limbs relaxed. Close your eyes. Imagine your next chemotherapy treatment and feel your body accepting the treatment without any problems: no nausea, no side effects. Feel the cancer cells dying and being flushed out of your body by your strong kidneys and powerful lungs.

Imagine the future, perhaps when this course of chemotherapy is complete. Imagine your body as stronger and healthier. Try to imagine this future in as much detail as possible.

Where are you and what are you doing? How does your body feel?

Imagine your muscles to be strong and all your senses alert.

Feel your mind become flexible and sharp.

Feel yourself grounded in your heart as it circulates your blood freely, nourishing you.

Stay in this future for a while, breathing in and out, feeling energized and alive.

CHAPTER 7

RECOVERY

FINISH LINE

Chemo is coming to an end. From now on, you won't be seeing your oncologist as often, and you no longer have a standing date with the chemo chair. Your immune system will start to improve, and your hair will start to grow back. You might feel joyful that you have crossed the finish line! Hurrah!

On the other hand, you might have a pang of sadness that your friends won't check on you as often or bring by lasagna now that "you're done." The calendar just opened up, and this unscheduled time might make you feel unsettled. You may be wondering about what happens next, now that this chemo triathlon is over. Imagining the future, you have probably just realized that *there is no finish line.*

After chemotherapy, there is no finish line for many reasons. You might need more treatment, such as radiation, surgery or even more chemotherapy. If you have advanced cancer that will be with you the rest of your life, chemotherapy may be an ongoing or recurrent part of your routine. Even if your chemo chapter is truly over, the experience is now and will forever be a part of you. The process of integrating cancer and what it means for you into the rest of your life is only beginning. Instead of feeling elated and ready to pop the champagne, you might be feeling disoriented and even a bit sad.

If that's how you're feeling, be assured that there is nothing wrong with you. The frenzy of getting it all done during active treatment provided a buffer from having to figure out what it all means. Once chemo is not occupying your time, you can begin to process your chemotherapy experience and see how cancer and chemo will impact the rest of your life.

INVISIBLE DAMAGE

The bald head, puffy face, swollen feet and discolored skin that chemo gives you are all visible side effects. As these symptoms resolve and you look more normal, you may feel that your outside is healing faster than your inside. There are many other common side effects that linger long after chemo is over, yet none are noticeable by other people. Do you still have nerve damage, foggy thinking or pain? What about anxiety or sadness? All the stress, fear and worry that you felt during chemotherapy and your other cancer treatments may have left you feeling lost. You may feel that you don't know who you are anymore. Feeling this way is extremely common.

Once you look "normal" again, it's easy for others around you to assume that you feel great and that chemotherapy is far behind you. In fact, you are still experiencing the emotional and physical fallout from treatment. Not only are you still feeling bad, but this disconnect between how people see you and how you experience yourself is very lonely. It can even feel like you are disconnected from life or living in a different reality.

You will feel less lonely if you can share how you are really doing

> ❤ **HELPFUL HINT**
>
> Not everyone who asks "How are you?" wants to hear the real answer, especially if the answer is "Not good!" Don't feel guilty about answering with "I'm fine" if you don't have the energy or don't feel like sharing the real answer.

with someone close to you. This could be a friend or loved one who helped you through your chemo experience, or it might be a fellow chemotherapy patient, such as someone in your support group. When you are ready, talk about how you really feel and what your body is experiencing. Don't feel pressured to meet anyone's expectations about getting better, including your own. You may be surprised at your real feelings: relief, anger, guilt or nothing. Observe what you feel without judging.

FALLOUT: LONG-TERM SIDE EFFECTS

Chemo may be over, but there are long-term side effects that are still around. You are not weak or defective if you can't bounce back to normal or jump back into your former life in a few weeks. It frequently takes up to a year to get your energy back, and some side effects, such as neuropathy, can take years to resolve. Here is a list of the most common problems that patients who have undergone chemotherapy commonly experience after treatment ends.

Post-Chemotherapy Long-Term Effects

- Anemia/low blood counts
- Body image difficulty
- Breathing difficulty/lung dysfunction
- Constipation and/or diarrhea
- Depression and anxiety
- Heart problems/heart failure
- Immune suppression
- Infertility
- Insomnia
- Memory problems or other brain dysfunction ("chemo brain")
- Nausea and other eating problems
- Neuropathy (nerve damage)
- Pain
- Osteoporosis (thin and weak bones)
- Sexual dysfunction, such as low sex drive, erectile dysfunction, vaginal dryness and pain, painful intercourse
- Skin and hair changes
- Swelling/lymphedema
- Urinary incontinence

It's such a long list. The first thing to do is to take a moment to notice if you are experiencing any of these symptoms. Then give yourself a break. You are still recovering, and you should permit yourself to stay in recovery mode. It can be frustrating to realize that recovery is going to take time and regaining your health and vigor will be another long road, just as chemotherapy was. Allow yourself to feel any anger or grief at this prospect—grief is a normal response. Treat yourself tenderly and return to caring for yourself with all the love that you did when you were undergoing treatment. You can use the techniques that worked for you during chemo to get you through this phase as well.

Prepare to manage any ongoing chemotherapy side effects by talking with your doctors and oncology treatment team. The next several sections dive into the details of many problems and how to manage them. Many of these symptoms and conditions will improve with time, and you can learn to manage them if you take a gentle and caring approach to yourself.

STILL SO TIRED: FATIGUE

Fatigue is the number one persistent side effect of chemotherapy. It may take you a year or more to recover your energy. You might feel frustrated or sad. You may miss the person you used to be or long for the things that you used to do.

Be patient and allow yourself time to recover. Trust in your ability to heal and to care for yourself. By using the strategies below, you can actively increase your energy during this healing period. Be persistent and you will discover what is best for you to relieve fatigue and increase your energy.

Strategies to Improve Energy

Exercise: Regular exercise has been shown to improve energy levels in people with cancer. Keep up the exercise you started during chemo or start a new routine of regular exercise. Build up slowly to avoid injury, and as you become stronger, you can increase your exercise intensity.

Sleep: Adults need between seven and eight hours of sleep per night. You may need more than this in the initial phase of recovery. Allow yourself enough time in bed for falling asleep and getting your hours of sleep. Discuss insomnia with your doctor if it takes you more than thirty minutes to fall asleep or if you wake frequently in the early morning hours.

Good Nutrition: Look at what you are eating and drinking. Are you drinking enough water? Dehydration causes fatigue. Are you eating too much sugar? The ups and downs of blood sugar can cause fatigue in the form of a "sugar crash." Return to eating protein at every meal and lots of vegetables and fruits, minimizing sugar and staying hydrated.

Consider Depression: Fatigue is one symptom of depression. Ask yourself if your mood is always down or if you have trouble enjoying the good parts of your life. Talk about this with your doctor and ask about seeing a therapist or taking a medication for depression.

Stress Management: As you return to your usual duties at work and at home, your stress level may increase. Stress is exhausting. What can you do to manage your stress? Can you return to your Mindset? What techniques can you use to lessen how anxious or tense you feel? Restart what helped during your treatment or try a new technique. Many medications can cause fatigue or sleepiness, so it's helpful to review your medications with your doctor and ask if any can be changed or if the dose can be moved to bedtime.

⚠ MEDICAL ALERT

Tell your doctor if you have thoughts of killing yourself. While thinking about or worrying about death is normal during chemo, thoughts of suicide are a sign of depression.

NUMB: ONGOING NEUROPATHY

Neuropathy (nerve damage) caused by chemotherapy affects between 40 percent and 60 percent of chemotherapy patients. Let me restate this astounding statistic: at some time, the majority of people who have chemotherapy have nerve damage! Because nerves take so long to heal compared to other organs in the body, the symptoms take longer to resolve. Symptoms of pain, numbness, cramping, tingling or weakness may be present for months or years after chemotherapy treatment is over. Most neuropathy improves, but it may worsen before it gets better. Reducing neuropathy symptoms is important for functioning at your best with the least pain possible.

Despite millions of dollars of research spending over decades, medical science has not been able to find an adequate treatment for chemotherapy-induced peripheral neuropathy (CIPN). Currently, the most effective treatment for chemotherapy-induced neuropathy pain is the prescription medication duloxetine (Cymbalta). The dose starts at 30mg daily and can be increased to 120mg daily. However, for most people, a dose of duloxetine 60mg achieves the most benefit with the least side effects. Other medications, such as gabapentin and pregabalin, which are prescribed for other types of neuropathy, have been studied for CIPN, but these medications have not been shown to be helpful for improving chemotherapy-induced neuropathy.

> ❤ **HELPFUL HINT**
>
> The most helpful treatment for chemo-induced neuropathy is prescription duloxetine 30–60mg daily. Also try acupuncture one–two treatments weekly for six–twelve weeks.

Other than duloxetine, exercise and acupuncture have been shown to improve symptoms of chemotherapy-induced peripheral neuropathy. Studies of acupuncture for CIPN show that it is effective for improving symptoms of pain and numbness. Exercise has also been shown to improve the symptoms of CIPN, so if you didn't already have enough reason to exercise, here's another one!

While the research evidence is less than for acupuncture, there are several over-the-counter supplements that have some research supporting their use to improve neuropathy symptoms. These include acetyl-L-carnitine, alpha-lipoic acid, curcumin, green tea and omega-3 fatty acids.

Consider Over-the-Counter Supplements

- acetyl-L-carnitine, 500mg twice daily
- alpha lipoic acid, 600mg three times daily
- curcumin, 500mg twice daily
- green tea extract, 250mg daily, approximately equal to four cups brewed tea daily
- omega-3 fatty acids (fish oil), 1000–2000mg daily

> ⚠ **MEDICAL ALERT**
>
> Do not take supplements during active chemo, since some can make chemo less effective, and some can make neuropathy worse.

To find help with some of the nerve dysfunction associated with neuropathy, seek out the help of a physical therapist or physical medicine and rehabilitation physician. Physical therapy can improve your balance and strength by training your healthy nerves and muscles to compensate for your deficits. You can function better, feel better and have less risk of falls or injuries. Some patients also find relief from pain and numbness by using other musculoskeletal techniques such as massage, topical anesthetic patches or creams, magnesium skin spray and warm packs.

> ❤ **HELPFUL HINT**
>
> For a detailed discussion of neuropathy prevention and treatment, please see "Chapter 2: Preventing and Treating Side Effects"

Neuropathy can be a vexing and disheartening side effect of chemo-therapy, causing multiple symptoms for a long time. By using multiple strategies and being persistent, you can work with your doctor to find a way to manage your symptoms and live life despite neuropathy.

RUNNING SCARED: ANXIETY

It won't surprise you to hear that ongoing anxiety is common after che-motherapy. According to a recent large review study, significant anxiety lingers in up to 20 percent of cancer survivors. Persistent anxiety is even more common after chemo than persistent depression, and some people can even develop post-traumatic stress disorder, or PTSD.

✏️ DEFINITION: PTSD

A form of anxiety in response to a prior trauma that manifests as anxiety with physical responses, such as sweating and racing pulse, heightened vigilance, nightmares, intrusive thoughts or flashbacks and avoidance of "triggers."

While not everyone develops PTSD, it is very normal to have an increase in anxiety around the time of follow-up doctor visits, tests or scans. This "scanxiety" and other routine worries can be effectively managed if you return to your stress-management routine. This could be exercise, meditation, prayer or humor. Reaching out to your cancer support community around the time of testing and scans is also very helpful for relieving scanxiety, since this is the tribe of people that knows best what you are going through. The more support you can get, the better, to help you return to playing your best mind game!

Occasionally, cancer-related anxiety requires more formal treat-ment, including prescription medication. If you have worry or distress that has any of the features listed below, discuss it with your doctor. You may benefit from attending a support group, meeting with a therapist or starting a medication.

Symptoms of Anxiety

- Worrying all the time
- Intrusive fearful thoughts or memories ("flashbacks") that interrupt your day
- Feeling "jumpy" all the time
- Constant fear of cancer recurrence
- Insomnia due to worry or not being able to "turn your mind off"
- Racing heartbeat, sweaty palms or butterflies in your stomach

Anxiety doesn't have to be permanent or disabling. There are ways to manage it and treat it, but first you need to recognize it. As always, listen to yourself, trust in your ability to heal and reach out for help.

BRITTLE BONES: OSTEOPOROSIS

You may have received steroids before or during chemo treatments to reduce nausea. You may have entered early menopause because of the aggressive nature of the chemotherapy drugs. You may still be taking hormone-blocking drugs, such as an aromatase inhibitor, to suppress any cancer cells that might have survived in your body. All these things can cause osteoporosis, a condition where the bones become weak, brittle and prone to fracture.

Your doctor can monitor the bones of your spine and hip for osteoporosis by ordering a bone density test called a DEXA scan. This test produces a numeric score for each body area scanned, such as the spine or hip, as well as an average score of bone density. This score then helps to predict your risk of fractures and is part of the information that your doctor uses to decide if you need to take medication to prevent fractures.

If you have mildly decreased bone density, this is called osteopenia, and your doctor will recommend weight-bearing exercise, vitamin D and sufficient dietary calcium intake. You will also need to repeat a DEXA scan every year or two to monitor your bone density. For osteopenia, most patients are not prescribed medication to strengthen their bones. However, each person's health and fracture risk is unique. You and your doctor should discuss the details of whether or not a medication for osteopenia is right for you.

If your bone density scan shows osteoporosis, or significant bone density loss, your doctor will most likely recommend some type of medication as part of your treatment. This may be in the form of an oral bisphosphonate, such as alendronate; an intravenous bisphosphonate, such as zoledronic acid; or another medication, such as denosumab, teriparatide or a calcitonin analog. Each medication has risks and benefits that extend beyond the benefit to your bones. For example, some studies have shown that zoledronic acid (brand names Zometa and Reclast) helps to prevent the reoccurrence of certain types of breast cancer. On the other hand, all of the bisphosphonates have a small risk of certain rare types of bone growths and fractures. You should discuss all the details with your doctor, and don't feel rushed into a decision about which medication to start.

Whether you have normal bone density, osteopenia or osteoporosis, weight-bearing exercise is important to prevent and treat bone loss. Exercise that is classified as "weight-bearing" is called such because it moves your body weight against the force of gravity and stimulates your bones to build up their internal structure and lay down more calcium. This type of movement is what prevents further bone loss and can even make them stronger. When choosing a weight-bearing exercise, think of walking, dancing, jogging, high-intensity interval training routines or yoga. Swimming and cycling, while great for aerobic conditioning, are not weight-bearing exercises. Most types of exercise that are done while standing are weight-bearing and will stimulate the bones of the spine, pelvis and hips.

Recommendations for daily vitamin D and calcium intake depend on your age and sex. Adults up to age 70 should take 600 IU of vitamin D daily, while adults 71 years and older should take 800 IU daily. Your oncologist may recommend a higher dose of vitamin D if you are deficient. You should try to get calcium from your diet, if possible, since studies show that calcium-rich foods, such as dairy products and green leafy vegetables, have many other health benefits. Recently, calcium supplements have been linked to other health problems, such as kidney stones and increased risk of heart disease, so if you take a calcium supplement, do not take more than the total recommended daily dose of calcium for you. The recommended calcium requirements are 1000mg/day for adults 19–50 years and men 51–70 years, 1200mg/day for women 51–70 years, and 1200mg/day for all adults 71 years and older.

Chemotherapy can take a toll on your bones. With your doctor, discuss your risk of osteoporosis in the larger context of your overall health, and develop a plan together for treating osteoporosis and preventing fractures. As you recover and move forward with building up your health in other areas, remember your skeleton that has been holding you up all this time—it may need some rebuilding too!

YOUR SEX LIFE (OR LACK THEREOF): SEXUAL DYSFUNCTION

By now, if you've spent any time in a cancer support group, whether in person or online, then you've probably talked a lot about sex. Cancer and its various treatments, chemotherapy included, can devastate your sex life, and this can contribute to relationship tension, depression and decreased quality of life. For most people, sex is an important part of life. Figuring out how to make sex enjoyable again after chemotherapy is key to feeling fully recovered.

Chemotherapy disrupts your sex life for several reasons. For most people, chemo interrupts hormones. Many chemo regimens include medications that are hormone blockers, such as leuprolide (Lupron) or tamoxifen. These medications block the action of estrogen and testosterone at the target organ in body, thus putting the body into a hormone-deprived state. This interruption in the functioning of the sex hormone system causes several symptoms, such as erectile dysfunction in men, vaginal dryness and pelvic pain in women and low libido (sex drive) for everyone.

Chemotherapy can also interrupt the sex hormones even if a hormone-blocker is not part of your chemo regimen. This happens in women when the ovaries are damaged by chemotherapy drugs and they stop producing estrogen. Menstrual cycles stop and a woman enters menopause prematurely. Chemo can also cause neuropathy that affects the pelvic nerves in both men and women, causing decreased sensation, difficulty with sexual arousal and problems reaching orgasm.

Chemo isn't the only culprit responsible for unwanted celibacy after cancer treatment. Physical changes from surgery can cause pain or

> ♥ **HELPFUL HINT**
>
> Starting the conversation about sex with your partner is often the most difficult step. It's worth it to gather the courage to say, "I'm having trouble with sex right now."

interfere with your ability to move. Or you may not feel confident about your body after cancer surgery. Tissue damage due to radiation treatments can have similar effects. In addition, many medications, such as anti-depressants, can cause low sex drive and sexual dysfunction.

In the face of such circumstances, what can you do to get your sexy on? Just as with most things in "cancerland," nothing can guarantee that your sex life will be exactly the same as it was before your diagnosis. However, by attending to your sexuality, you can decrease pain and discomfort and improve how you feel about your body. This will help you regain intimacy with your partner or have the confidence to meet a new partner.

If you are currently in an intimate relationship, start by telling your partner that you are struggling with sex. This may be the most difficult step. When you show up and say that you are not in the mood, feeling pain during sex or can't "perform" in some other way, this is a point of maximum emotional vulnerability, but it's worth it. It's a starting point for discussion and improvement. You may consider visiting a counselor to help you sort through these topics, either on your own or with your partner. Many of the large cancer centers have counselors and therapists specifically dedicated to sexual health, so ask your oncologist or cancer survivorship treatment team about these services.

> ❤ **HELPFUL HINT**
>
> Exercise improves your sex life! Don't feel guilty about the days that you don't exercise, but instead feel proud of yourself on days when you do!

Since medications can interfere with sexual functioning, discuss your physical symptoms with your oncologist and review each medication that you are taking. Some medications, such as ongoing chemotherapy or other anti-cancer drugs, will be necessary and non-negotiable. However, if there is a medication that is causing a sexual side effect, such as erectile dysfunction or low libido, and the medication can be stopped or changed, then by all means it's worth trying to see if the side effect goes away!

Exercise has been mentioned many times, but it really is true: exercise is beneficial. Studies have shown that for cancer survivors, exercise improves your health in general and your sex life specifically. Keep making an effort to add regular exercise into your routine. Eventually you will get stronger and you'll find types of exercise that fit your level of health and fitness.

For men struggling with erectile dysfunction (ED), there are many prescription medications now on the market that improve the hardness and duration of erections. The most common medications in this class include sildenafil (Viagra), vardenafil (Staxyn and Levitra) and tadalafil (Cialis). Tadalafil can be taken daily at a low dose, and the others are taken shortly before intercourse. Unfortunately, most drugs to treat ED are not covered by medical insurance, but you can make the cost more affordable by asking your doctor to prescribe the highest dose and using a pill cutter to split the pills.

> **⚠ MEDICAL ALERT**
>
> Do not order erectile dysfunction medications (Viagra and similar) from online or foreign pharmacies, since these sources frequently sell medications that are fake or tainted with dangerous chemicals.

For women who have vaginal symptoms due to premature menopause or hormone-blocking drugs, there are several treatment options that can provide some relief. The most effective relief is taking hormone-replacement therapy, such as with an estrogen patch or pill, or combined estrogen-progesterone treatment. You can only use systemic hormone replacement therapy if your cancer was not hormone-related. Breast cancer and most gynecologic cancers are not compatible with using hormone replacement therapy.

If you can't take hormone replacement for vaginal tightness and pain, vaginal dilators are another option. Dilators gently stretch vaginal tissue and are used with a glycerin-based lubricant. There are several types of vaginal dilators, and some models automatically expand. For vaginal dryness, *Replens* is a long-lasting vaginal moisturizer specially designed for use after menopause, and it's available without a prescription at drug stores and grocery stores. Vaginal estrogen creams and suppositories are available by prescription and are excellent for restoring vaginal elasticity and moisture. However, whether or not you can use vaginal estrogen products depends on if you had a hormone-dependent cancer, such as ovarian or breast cancer. You should ask your oncologist if vaginal estrogen is a possible option for you. Most importantly, for more comfortable sex, always use a lubricant and lots of it!

In addition to topical moisturizers and estrogen creams, there is evidence that new types of laser treatments to the vagina, such as the MonaLisa® Touch by Cynosure, can help symptoms of vaginal and vulvar pain, tightness and dryness. Laser treatments are more invasive than a medication, so you should ask about side effects and only have procedures performed in a physician's office.

Remember that setting the stage for good sex is important—lighting candles, putting on music, giving your partner a massage or whatever else gets you both in the mood. Set aside enough time for intimacy that isn't sexual: talking, connecting and snuggling. Reconnecting emotionally with your partner doesn't have to be done right before jumping into bed–in fact, it may work better if you steal small moments of intimacy throughout the week, not just on date night.

Remember also that even if you don't have a partner, you can still get busy on your own! Masturbation isn't mandatory, but it is normal, and you may even learn something about what turns you on. Finally, think about expanding your ideas about what makes for good sexual foreplay, solo sex or the main event. Here's a list of resources for information and tools to get your juices flowing.

Personal Lubricants

- Astroglide at **https://astroglide.com/**
- Almost Naked Organic Personal Lubricant at **https://goodclean-love.com/products/almost-naked-organic-personal-lubricant**

- Isabel Fay Natural Water-Based Lubricant at Amazon, Walmart and at **http://www.lubeforever.com/**
- Replens Long-Lasting Vaginal Moisturizer at **http://replens.com/**
- Sliquid at **https://sliquid.com/**

Vaginal Dilators & Vibrators

- Eva vibrator at **https://www.dameproducts.com/**
- Milli Expanding Vaginal Dilator at **https://www.millimedical.com/**
- Doc Johnson The Original Pocket Rocket—Targeted Clitoral Massager
- Osé vibrator by Lora DeCarlo at **https://loradicarlo.com/**
- VIBIO Active Dilators Set Kegel Exerciser with Powered Handle and 4 Graduated Tips
- The Womanizer vibrator at **https://www.womanizer.com/us/**

Information Resources about Sexuality after Cancer Treatment

- Center for Intimacy after Cancer Therapy at **http://renewintimacy.org/**
- Information for Men on Sexual Wellbeing after Pelvic Cancer Treatment (booklet) at **https://www.hse.ie/eng/services/list/5/cancer/profinfo/resources/booklets/pelvic%20cancer.pdf**
- Sexual Wellbeing after Breast or Pelvic Cancer Treatment (booklet) at **https://www.hse.ie/eng/services/list/5/cancer/patient/leaflets/sexual-wellbeing-after-breast-or-pelvic-cancer-treatment.pdf**

Sex is deeply personal yet intimately shared. Know that you are not alone if you struggle with sexuality after your ordeal with cancer treatment. Regardless of how much sex you have, either with or without a partner, be confident that with some research, trial and error, and a sense of adventure, you can reclaim your sex life after chemotherapy.

CHASING THE HOLY GRAIL: PAIN CONTROL

Pain may be one of the lingering problems that you are faced with as you heal from the aftermath of your chemotherapy or live with ongoing cancer treatment. Pain interferes with sleep, work and enjoying life. Pain is one of the invisible symptoms that can be hard to quantify, difficult to explain to others and difficult to treat, especially since pain medications often cause other side effects. However, the better you can manage your pain, the better you will function and the better your quality of life.

If you have significant pain, make sure that you follow up with your oncologist to investigate the cause of the pain. One rule of thumb is that any new pain (or symptom) that has been present for two weeks needs to be discussed with your doctor. This allows your oncologist to investigate the cause of the pain and decide if any tests are needed. An old problem, such as nerve damage in your hands from chemo or an area of previously diagnosed tumor, may not necessarily prompt any new testing.

❤ HELPFUL HINT

Narcotics, duloxetine and gabapentin all cause constipation. If you take these medications for pain, take a daily regimen to prevent constipation, such as polyethylene glycol (Miralax) or prescription lactulose. Bisacodyl tablets can be taken a few times per week to help you have a bowel movement.

Narcotics, such as morphine, hydrocodone and oxycodone, are important for treating chronic cancer pain, but many other non-addictive medications are also effective to treat pain. These include medications that act on nerves, such as duloxetine and gabapentin; muscle relaxants, such as cyclobenzaprine; and non-steroidal anti-inflammatory drugs, such as naproxen and ibuprofen.

The most effective way to manage pain is a multi-pronged approach that addresses its many causes and uses a combination of medication and non-medication pain relief methods. For some people, referral to a pain-management specialist is a good option. Non-medication methods for pain control include things such as massage, heat and cold therapy, stretching, exercise, acupuncture, meditation and mindfulness-based stress reduction. Review your current pain medications and other pain management methods with your doctor, and together you can identify what can be done to get you successful pain relief.

⚠ **MEDICAL ALERT**

With the increase in opioid addiction in the US, treatment of chronic pain has come under greater regulation. Cancer patients may have trouble getting prescriptions for some types of narcotic pain relievers. Keep up with your appointments and refills to avoid running out of medication.

FINANCIAL TOXICITY

The cost of cancer treatment is huge. Most of you have likely spent a small fortune trying to reclaim your health from cancer, not even including the time lost from work and other activities. This is especially true for people who live in the United States and other countries that lack universal health care coverage. The long-term side effect of the high cost of cancer treatment has been termed financial toxicity, and it can be devastating.

There are resources available to assist with the financial burden of treatment. First, if you cannot work because of your diagnosis, you may qualify for a disability income program. In the United States, the disability income program is Supplemental Security Income (SSI). For assistance during treatment, many organizations have grants and programs available to assist people with paying for their cancer-related care, as do several pharmaceutical companies. This list is a starting place to find financial and legal help.

Resources for Financial Advice and Assistance

- Cancer Council (Australia) at **https://www.cancer.org.au/**
- Cancer Legal Resource Center at **https://thedrlc.org/cancer/**
- Cancer Support Community—Managing the Cost of Cancer Treatment at **https://www.cancersupportcommunity.org/ living-cancer-topics/managing-cost-cancer-treatment**
- Cancer and Work (Canada) at **https://www.cancerandwork.ca/**
- Chemocare—Financial Assistance at **http://chemocare.com/ chemotherapy/before-and-after/financial-assistance-programs.aspx**
- Macmillan Cancer Support (United Kingdom) at **https://www.macmillan.org.uk/**
- PAN Foundation for financial assistance at **https://panfoundation.org/index.php/en/**

- Young Survival Coalition—Financial Assistance at https://www.youngsurvival.org/learn/living-with-breast-cancer/practical-concerns/financial-assistance
- Supplemental Security Income (SSI) at https://www.ssa.gov/ssi/index.htm

EXPLORE HOW YOU REALLY FEEL

Now that you've discovered that the mind game doesn't end when chemo ends, it's more important than ever to take care of your mental health. If you haven't already been writing or journaling as you've been going through treatment, it's not too late to start. A journal is a private place for you to vent your frustrations, note any feelings and record how those feelings—and your body—change over time.

Another safe place to explore your feelings is within a support group of cancer survivors. It's worth noting that many support groups are designated as either for early-stage disease or for metastatic/advanced disease. It's debatable whether or not this division is a good thing, since some people believe that all those who have experienced cancer can learn from each other regardless of stage and regardless of whether their cancer is in remission or not. You may have to try a few groups before you find a group that feels right for you and where you feel safe to voice your true feelings.

If you are really struggling emotionally or if you are depressed, see a counselor or psychologist. Individual therapy is private, non-biased and focused on your best interests. Ask your doctor to refer you to a licensed counselor, or seek out mental health professionals through your medical insurance plan, preferably someone who has worked with cancer patients in recovery.

If you prefer an online forum, visit the website for the Invisible Disabilities Association (**https://www.invisibledisabilities.org**) for ideas and support. This group's mission is to increase awareness about invisible illness, pain and disabilities, and to encourage and educate people affected by such issues. Reading blog posts from other cancer survivors can also be helpful. The website IHadCancer (**https://www.ihadcancer. com/**) publishes a variety of blog posts written by cancer patients and survivors. Facebook, Instagram and Twitter also manage groups that focus on cancer survivorship and recovery. To get a feel for what's happening in these online communities, join a group or two and listen in for a while. Once you have a sense of the culture of the group, it's your choice whether to stay and participate or not.

Resources for Recovery after Chemotherapy and Cancer

- GRYT Health at **https://grythealth.com/**
- IHadCancer at **https://www.ihadcancer.com/**
- Invisible Disabilities Association at **https://invisibledisabilities.org/**
- National Coalition for Cancer Survivorship at **https://www.canceradvocacy.org/**
- Young Survival Coalition at **http://blog.youngsurvival.org/cancer-ever-after/**

Regardless of how you do it, keep an eye on your inner self. Remember that the mind game continues long after the chemotherapy stops. To keep yourself healthy, strong and in the game, honor your real feelings and find a community that supports you.

ONWARD

You have overcome so much. You have been so brave, continuing chemotherapy in the face of fear and exhaustion, pain and loss. It would have been so much easier to give up, to slide into surrender and lose yourself. But you didn't. You're here. Let's recap everything that you did for yourself.

During chemotherapy you . . .

- became an expert in your disease and in yourself
- prepared gear and supplies for home and for treatment days at the clinic
- asked for advice from loved ones
- accepted strong drugs into your body and asked them to help heal you
- ate food to fuel yourself, even when you weren't hungry
- thought that your bones were going to break from pain
- held your tongue even when you wanted to scream
- screamed at someone when you didn't mean it
- realized that you are fragile and asked for help
- slept for longer than you thought was possible
- looked Death in the eye
- fell apart over and over because it seemed too hard
- picked yourself up every single time because you knew that it was worth it
- decided to ignore the things that just aren't important

- realized that you are strong, much stronger than you realized
- realized that you are brave

I'm sure that there is so much more that needs to be on this list of what you have done. If you are inspired, take a pen right now, and keep adding to the list. You can refer to it often, to remind you of where you've been and what you've accomplished. As a final exercise, use this visualization to tune in with the part of yourself that is steady and sure, untouched by illness or the ravages of chemo.

Anchor to Your Core

Take a moment to feel that part of you that is untouched by illness. Visualize your healthy core that chemo has not stolen, that side effects have not damaged.

This is your vibrant and infinite self.

There is no fear or disease that can touch you here, at your core.

This true center is strong and yet fragile. Be tender with yourself.

Anchor yourself to this thriving core and look ahead.

Feel your strength, as you are braving onward, braving life.

STAY IN TOUCH

For additional chemotherapy tips, bonus materials and Braving Chemo updates, sign up on my website: **BeverlyZavaletaMD.com** (**https://www. beverlyzavaletamd.com/**)

You can also keep in touch by following me on Twitter and Instagram at @BZavaletaMD

BIBLIOGRAPHY & RESOURCES

General Cancer Information and Cancer Resources

6 Incredibly Useful Apps for Cancer Patients. (n.d.). Retrieved February 10, 2018, from TheSocialMedwork website: http://thesocialmedwork.com/blog/cancer-patient-tech-apps

A Patient's Guide to Navigating the Insurance Appeals Process. (n.d.). Retrieved February 8, 2018, from http://www.patientadvocate.org/requests/publications/Guide-Appeals-Process.pdf

Breast Advocate® App. (n.d.). Retrieved August 7, 2019, from Breast Advocate® App website: https://breastadvocateapp.com

Cancer Council Australia. Cancer information and support. Retrieved September 4, 2019, from https://www.cancer.org.au/

Cancer and Work. (n.d.). Retrieved August 14, 2019, from Cancer and Work website: https://www.cancerandwork.ca/

Cancercare.org, Cancer Support Groups, Counseling, Education, Publications, Financial Assistance. (n.d.). Retrieved January 25, 2018, from CancerCare website: https://www.cancercare.org/

Cancercenters.cancer.gov. (n.d.). Retrieved January 25, 2018, from https://cancercenters.cancer.gov/

Cancer Survival Toolbox. (n.d.). Retrieved February 10, 2018, from NCCS - National Coalition for Cancer Survivorship website: https://www.canceradvocacy.org/resources/cancer-survival-toolbox

Cancer-treatment-and-survivorship-facts-and-figures-2016-2017.pdf. (n.d.). Retrieved from https://www.cancer.org/content/dam/cancer-org/research/cancer-facts-and-statistics/cancer-treatment-and-survivorship-facts-and-figures/cancer-treatment-and-survivorship-facts-and-figures-2016-2017.pdf

CareZone | Easily organize health information in one place. (n.d.). Retrieved February 10, 2018, from https://carezone.com/home

CaringBridge Personal Health Journals for Recovery, Cancer & More. (n.d.). Retrieved February 16, 2018, from CaringBridge website: https://www.caringbridge.org/

Drake, E. (2015, August 26). 5 Things You May Not Know About Oncofertility. Retrieved February 10, 2018, from Huffington Post website: https://www.huffingtonpost.com/emily-drake/5-things-you-should-know-about-oncofertility_b_8037942.html

Eva | A mobile app for peer to peer cancer support. (n.d.). Retrieved July 27, 2019, from http://www.eva-app.co/

Girard, V. (2008). *There's No Place Like Hope: A Guide to Beating Cancer in Mind-Sized Bites* (1 edition; D. Zadra, Ed.). Compendium Publishing & Communications.

Guide2chemo.com. (2014, March 4). Retrieved February 20, 2018, from http://guide2chemo.com/chemo-basics

How to appeal an insurance company decision. (n.d.). Retrieved February 8, 2018, from HealthCare.gov website: https://www.healthcare.gov/appeal-insurance-company-decision/appeals/

IHadCancer.com. (n.d.-a). Cancer Support Community for Peer to Peer Help |... Retrieved July 25, 2019, from https://www.ihadcancer.com/

Live Better With Cancer. (n.d.). Retrieved July 13, 2019, from Live Better With Cancer website: https://cancer.livebetterwith.com/

Living With App | This Is Living With Cancer | Official Site. (n.d.). Retrieved August 16, 2019, from https://www.thisislivingwithcancer.com/living-with-app

McKay, J., & MSN, T. S. R. O. (2009). *The Chemotherapy Survival Guide: Everything You Need to Know to Get Through Treatment* (3rd edition). Oakland, Calif: New Harbinger Publications.

My Lifeline: Cancer support, free personal cancer patient websites and blogs, information about cancer treatment, and being a patient caregiver. (n.d.). Retrieved April 25, 2019, from MyLifeLine website: https://www.mylifeline.org/

National Cancer Institute. (n.d.). Retrieved January 25, 2018, from https://www.cancer.gov/

Navigating Care. (n.d.). Retrieved February 16, 2018, from http://www.navigatingcare.com/patient/

NCCN - Evidence-Based Cancer Guidelines, Oncology Drug Compendium, Oncology Continuing Medical Education. (n.d.). Retrieved February 15, 2018, from https://www.nccn.org/

Oncolink. (n.d.). Retrieved February 10, 2018, from https://www.oncolink.org/

Patient Advocate Foundation. (n.d.). Retrieved February 8, 2018, from http://patientadvocate.org/

Peries, A. (2018). *Chemo Journal: Chemotherapy Treatment Cycle Tracker, Side Effects Journal & Medical Appointments Diary| Size 8" x 10"|Discreet Christian Cover Notebook.* CreateSpace Independent Publishing Platform.

Pocket Cancer Care Guide. (n.d.). Retrieved February 10, 2018, from NCCS - National Coalition for Cancer Survivorship website: https://www.canceradvocacy.org/resources/pocket-care-guide/

Rethink Breast Cancer. (2015, August 23). Retrieved February 9, 2018, from Rethink Breast Cancer website: https://rethinkbreastcancer.com/news/

Ride Health. (n.d.). Retrieved August 22, 2019, from Ride Health website: https://www.ride-health.com

Robin Care. (n.d.). Retrieved September 3, 2019, from Robin Care website: https://www.robincare.com/

SignUpGenius.com: Free Online Sign Up Forms. (n.d.). Retrieved September 3, 2019, from https://www.signupgenius.com/

Stupid Cancer. (n.d.). Retrieved June 26, 2019, from Stupid Cancer website: https://stupidcancer.org/

Teen Cancer America—Resources. (n.d.). Retrieved April 24, 2019, from Teen Cancer America website: https://teencanceramerica.org/news-resources/resources/

The State of Cancer Care in America, 2017: A Report by the American Society of Clinical Oncology. (2017). *Journal of Oncology Practice, 13*(4), e353–e394. https://doi.org/10.1200/JOP.2016.020743

Tigerlily Foundation for Breast Cancer. (2016, August 5). Retrieved June 26, 2019, from Tigerlily Foundation website: https://www.tigerlilyfoundation.org/about-us/

Wellness Link for Kris Carr, New York Times best-selling author and wellness activist. (n.d.). Retrieved July 15, 2019, from KrisCarr.com website: https://kriscarr.com/

Young Survival Coalition. (n.d.). Retrieved May 29, 2018, from Young Survival Coalition, Young women facing breast cancer together. website: https://www.youngsurvival.org/learn/about-breast-cancer/statistics

Books

A Patient's Guide to Navigating the Insurance Appeals Process. (n.d.). Retrieved February 8, 2018, from **http://www.patientadvocate.org/requests/publications/Guide-Appeals-Process.pdf**

Beattie, M. (1996). *Journey to the Heart: Daily Meditations on the Path to Freeing Your Soul* (1st edition). San Francisco, Calif.: HarperSanFrancisco.

Besser, J., & Grant, B. L. (2019). *What to eat during cancer treatment* (Second edition). Altanta, GA: American Cancer Society.

BJ Miller MD, & Berger, S. (2019). *A Beginner's Guide to the End.* Simon & Schuster.

Bowler, K. (2018). *Everything happens for a reason: And other lies I've loved.* New York: Random House.

Brach, T. (2016). *True Refuge: Finding Peace and Freedom in Your Own Awakened Heart* (Reprint edition). New York: Bantam.

Brown, B. (2010). *The Gifts of Imperfection: Let Go of Who You Think You're Supposed to Be and Embrace Who You Are* (1 edition). Center City, Minn: Hazelden Publishing.

Brown, R., Mastej, B., & M.D, J. S. L. (2011). *Chemo: Secrets to Thriving: From someone who's been there.* (1st edition). Bedford, IN: Norlightspress.Com.

Burch, V., Penman, D., & Williams, M. (2015). *You Are Not Your Pain: Using Mindfulness to Relieve Pain, Reduce Stress, and Restore Well-Being---An Eight-Week Program* (Unabridged edition). New York; Prince Frederick, MD: Macmillan Audio.

Chodron, P. (2016). *When Things Fall Apart: Heart Advice for Difficult Times* (Anniversary edition). Boulder, Colorado: Shambhala.

Connell, W., & Connell, S. (2014). *But You LOOK Good: How to Encourage and Understand People Living with Illness and Pain.* Invisible Disabilities Association.

Gawande, A. (2017). *Being Mortal: Medicine and What Matters in the End.* Picador USA.

Girard, V. (2008). *There's No Place Like Hope: A Guide to Beating Cancer in Mind-Sized Bites* (1 edition; D. Zadra, Ed.). Compendium Publishing & Communications.

Goldstein, K. M., Coeytaux, R. R., Williams, J. W., Shepherd-Banigan, M., Goode, A. P., McDuffie, J. R., … Wing, L. (2016). *Nonpharmacologic Treatments for*

Menopause-Associated Vasomotor Symptoms. Retrieved from http://www.ncbi.nlm.nih.gov/books/NBK447618/

Kabat-Zinn, J. (2005). *Wherever You Go, There You Are: Mindfulness Meditation in Everyday Life* (10 edition). New York: Hachette Books.

Katz, R., & Edelson, M. (2017). *The Cancer-Fighting Kitchen, Second Edition: Nourishing, Big-Flavor Recipes for Cancer Treatment and Recovery* (Revised ed. edition). Berkeley: Ten Speed Press.

Lamott, A. (2012). *Help, Thanks, Wow: The Three Essential Prayers* (First Printing edition). New York: Riverhead Books.

McKay, J., & MSN, T. S. R. O. (2009). *The Chemotherapy Survival Guide: Everything You Need to Know to Get Through Treatment* (3rd edition). Oakland, Calif: New Harbinger Publications.

Nhất Hạnh. (2008). The Miracle of Mindfulness. London: Rider.

Piver, S. (2015). *Start Here Now: An Open-Hearted Guide to the Path and Practice of Meditation*. Boston: Shambhala.

Servan-Schreiber MD PhD, D. (2017). *Anticancer: A New Way of Life* (Reprint edition). Penguin Books.

Trent, J. D. (2019). *Dessert First: Preparing for Death While Savoring Life*. Chalice Press.

Side Effect Management

Acupuncture Find a Practitioner Directory | NCCAOM. (n.d.). Retrieved February 8, 2018, from **http://www.nccaom.org/find-a-practitioner-directory/**

Acupuncture. (2011, December 1). Retrieved February 8, 2018, from NCCIH website: ***https://nccih.nih.gov/health/acupuncture***

Alliance for Fertility Preservation | Fertility Preservation for Cancer Patients. (n.d.). Retrieved July 25, 2019, from **https://www.allianceforfertilitypreservation.org/index.htm**

Almost Naked Organic Personal Lubricant. (n.d.). Retrieved August 14, 2019, from Good Clean Love website: **https://goodcleanlove.com/products/almost-naked-organic-personal-lubricant**

ASTROGLIDE Personal Lubricant. (n.d.). Products | Retrieved August 14, 2019, from Astroglide website: **https://www.astroglide.com/products/**

Burch, V., Penman, D., & Williams, M. (2015). *You Are Not Your Pain: Using Mindfulness to Relieve Pain, Reduce Stress, and Restore Well-Being—An Eight-Week Program* (Unabridged edition). New York; Prince Frederick, MD: Macmillan Audio.

CDC—Information for Health Care Providers About Preventing Infections in Cancer Patients. (2017, October 25). Retrieved March 5, 2018, from https://www.cdc.gov/cancer/preventinfections/providers.htm

The Center for Intimacy after Cancer, CIACT, Inc., Helping change the quality of life and renew intimacy after cancer treatment. (n.d.). Retrieved August 14, 2019, from http://www.renewintimacy.org/

Connell, W., & Connell, S. (2014). *But You LOOK Good: How to Encourage and Understand People Living with Illness and Pain.* Invisible Disabilities Association.

Gem Gem's Ginger Candy. (n.d.). Retrieved February 7, 2018, from http://www.gemgemsweet.com/about.en

Gin Gins® Original Chewy Ginger Candy. (n.d.). Retrieved February 7, 2018, from https://gingerpeople.com/products/gin-gins-original-chewy-ginger-candy/

Ginger Honey Tea. (n.d.). Retrieved February 8, 2018, from Food Network website: https://www.foodnetwork.com/recipes/rachael-ray/ginger-honey-tea-recipe-1917101

Infection Prevention from CDC. (2017, October 27). Retrieved March 5, 2018, from https://www.cdc.gov/cancer/preventinfections/patients.htm

Information for Men on Sexual Wellbeing After Pelvic Cancer Treatment. (n.d.). Retrieved from https://www.hse.ie/eng/services/list/5/cancer/profinfo/resources/booklets/pelvic%20cancer.pdf

Invisible Disabilities Association—IDA - Encourage | Educate | Connect | Invisible No More. (n.d.). Retrieved January 25, 2018, from Invisible Disabilities Association—IDA website: https://invisibledisabilities.org/

LookGoodFeelBetter. (n.d.). Retrieved January 25, 2018, from Look Good Feel Better website: http://lookgoodfeelbetter.org/

MetaQil | Metallic Taste in Mouth Remedy | Instant Relief. (n.d.). Retrieved September 3, 2019, from https://metaqil.com/

Murphy, H., McCarthy, T., Lyng, A., Doherty, K., Mullen, L., & Bonas, F. (2018). Sexual Well-Being After Breast or Pelvic Cancer Treatment: A Guide for Women. *Journal of Global Oncology,* (4_suppl_2), 179s–179s. https://doi.org/10.1200/jgo.18.68000

The Rapunzel Project® > Home. (n.d.). Retrieved February 9, 2018, from http://rapunzelproject.org/

Replens Comfort Gel. Daily External Vaginal Moisturizer | Retrieved August 14, 2019, from Replens Long-Lasting Vaginal Moisturizer website: http://www.replens.com/Products/Replens-Moisture-Restore-External-Comfort-Gel/

Hair Loss Prevention and Management

Headcovers | Chemo Headwear | Cancer Headwear (n.d.). Retrieved July 13, 2019, from https://www.headcovers.com/headwear/

Make a Wig From Your Own Hair. (n.d.). Retrieved July 23, 2019, from Compassionate Creations Wig Design website: https://compassionatecreationswigdesign.com/make-a-wig-from-your-own-hair/

Paxman Scalp Cooling. (n.d.). Retrieved February 9, 2018, from Paxman USA website: https://www.paxmanusa.com

Penguin Cold Caps. (n.d.). Retrieved February 9, 2018, from Penguin Cold Caps website: https://penguincoldcaps.com/us/

Scalp Cooling System from Dignitana | Cold Caps | Chemotherapy Hair Loss. (n.d.). Retrieved February 9, 2018, from Dignicap website: https://dignicap.com/

The Rapunzel Project® > Home. (n.d.). Retrieved February 9, 2018, from http://rapunzelproject.org/

Exercise

An Overview of Physical Therapy Exercises. Retrieved June 17, 2019, from Verywell Health website: https://www.verywellhealth.com/physical-therapy-exercises-4013311

Bailey, T. G., Cable, N. T., Aziz, N., Atkinson, G., Cuthbertson, D. J., Low, D. A., & Jones, H. (2016). Exercise training reduces the acute physiological severity of post-menopausal hot flushes. *The Journal of Physiology*, *594*(3), 657–667. https://doi.org/10.1113/JP271456

Daley, A., Stokes-Lampard, H., Thomas, A., & MacArthur, C. (2014). Exercise for vasomotor menopausal symptoms. In *Cochrane Database of Systematic Reviews*. https://doi.org/10.1002/14651858.CD006108.pub4

DoYogaWithMe.com Free Online Yoga Videos—Classes and Poses | DoYogaWithMe.com. (n.d.). Retrieved January 25, 2018, from https://www.doyogawithme.com/

Exercising During Cancer Treatment. (n.d.). Retrieved February 15, 2018, from https://www.nccn.org/patients/resources/life_with_cancer/exercise.aspx

Gaia—Conscious Media, Yoga & More. (n.d.). Retrieved January 25, 2018, from Gaia website: https://www.gaia.com

Glo Inc, (n.d.). | Unlimited access to yoga, meditation, and Pilates classes. Retrieved July 23, 2019, from https://www.glo.com/

MoveforwardPT.com Cancer Page. (2017, February 1). Retrieved February 15, 2018, from American Physical Therapy Association website: https://www.moveforwardpt.com/SymptomsConditionsDetail. aspx?cid=256fdb5e-efde-44db-bbb3-ca2d56e68b50

Servan-Schreiber MD PhD, D. (2017). *Anticancer: A New Way of Life* (Reprint edition). Penguin Books.

Tai Chi for Health Institute Dr. Paul Lam. (n.d.). Retrieved February 21, 2018, from Tai Chi for Health Institute website: https://taichiforhealthinstitute.org/what-is-tai-chi/

Nutrition

Besser, J., Ratley, K., Knecht, S., & Szafranski, M. (2009). *What to Eat During Cancer Treatment: 100 Great-Tasting, Family-Friendly Recipes to Help You Cope* (1 edition). Atlanta, GA: American Cancer Society.

Foodsafety.gov. (n.d.). Recalls & Alerts. Retrieved February 19, 2018, from https://www.foodsafety.gov/recalls/index.html

Healthy Living App (by EWG). Retrieved February 20, 2018, from https://www.ewg.org/apps

Katz, R., & Edelson, M. (2017). *The Cancer-Fighting Kitchen, Second Edition: Nourishing, Big-Flavor Recipes for Cancer Treatment and Recovery* (Revised ed. edition). Berkeley: Ten Speed Press.

Recommended Nutrition Books—Dana-Farber Cancer Institute | Boston, MA. (n.d.). Retrieved July 17, 2019, from https://www.dana-farber.org/health-library/articles/recommended-nutrition-books/

Servan-Schreiber MD PhD, D. (2017). *Anticancer: A New Way of Life* (Reprint edition). Penguin Books.

Soluble Fiber Primer—Plus the Top Five Foods That Can Lower LDL Cholesterol. (n.d.). Retrieved February 9, 2018, from http://www.todaysdietitian.com/newarchives/120913p16.shtml

Mindfulness, Relaxation, Insomnia and Sleep

Beattie, M. (1996). *Journey to the Heart: Daily Meditations on the Path to Freeing Your Soul* (1st edition). San Francisco, Calif.: HarperSanFrancisco.

Bodhi Mind Meditation App—A Path to Awakening—On Your iPhone. (n.d.). Retrieved July 23, 2019, from https://www.bodhimind.me/

Brach, T. (2016). *True Refuge: Finding Peace and Freedom in Your Own Awakened Heart* (Reprint edition). New York: Bantam.

Breathe2Relax | t2health. (n.d.). Retrieved June 4, 2017, from http://t2health.dcoe.mil/apps/breathe2relax

Breathing Exercise: Three To Try | 4-7-8 Breath | Andrew Weil, M.D. (n.d.). Retrieved February 11, 2018, from https://www.drweil.com/health-wellness/body-mind-spirit/stress-anxiety/breathing-three-exercises/

Burch, V., Penman, D., & Williams, M. (2015). *You Are Not Your Pain: Using Mindfulness to Relieve Pain, Reduce Stress, and Restore Well-Being---An Eight-Week Program* (Unabridged edition). New York; Prince Frederick, MD: Macmillan Audio.

Calm. (n.d.-a). Retrieved September 17, 2019, from https://www.calm.com

Chodron, P. (2016). *When Things Fall Apart: Heart Advice for Difficult Times* (Anniversary edition). Boulder, Colorado: Shambhala.

Free Guided Meditations—UCLA Mindful Awareness Research Center—Los Angeles, CA. (n.d.). Retrieved February 20, 2018, from http://marc.ucla.edu/mindful-meditations

Gaia—Conscious Media, Yoga & More. (n.d.). Retrieved January 25, 2018, from Gaia website: https://www.gaia.com

Glo | Unlimited access to yoga, meditation, and Pilates classes. Retrieved July 23, 2019, from https://www.glo.com/

Hanh, T. N. (1999). *The Miracle of Mindfulness: An Introduction to the Practice of Meditation* (1st edition; M. Ho, Trans.). Princeton, N.J.: Beacon Press.

Healthy_sleep.pdf. (n.d.). Retrieved from https://www.nhlbi.nih.gov/files/docs/public/sleep/healthy_sleep.pdf

Insight Timer Meditation Timer. Retrieved January 25, 2018, from https://insighttimer.com

Kabat-Zinn, J. (2005). *Wherever You Go, There You Are: Mindfulness Meditation in Everyday Life* (10 edition). New York: Hachette Books.

Kundalini Breathing Pranayam Techniques. (n.d.). Retrieved February 18, 2018, from 3HO - Happy, Healthy, Holy website: https://www.3ho.org/kundalini-yoga/pranayam/pranayam-techniques

Lamott, A. (2012). *Help, Thanks, Wow: The Three Essential Prayers* (First Printing edition). New York: Riverhead Books.

Mindful.org Meditation. (n.d.). Retrieved June 4, 2017, from
https://www.mindful.org/meditation/

Mrs.Mindfulness.com. (n.d.). Retrieved February 20, 2018, from Mrs. Mindfulness
website: https://mrsmindfulness.com/

National Sleep Foundation—Sleep Research & Education. (n.d.). Retrieved
February 10, 2018, from https://sleepfoundation.org/

Open Heart Project. (n.d.). Retrieved February 20, 2018, from Susan Piver website:
https://susanpiver.com/open-heart-project/

Piver, S. (2015). *Start Here Now: An Open-Hearted Guide to the Path and Practice of
Meditation.* Boston: Shambhala.

Understanding the stress response. Retrieved January 25, 2018,
from Harvard Health Publishing, H. H. (n.d.). website:
https://www.health.harvard.edu/staying-healthy/understanding-the-stress-response

Sleep Disorders [PdqCancerInfoSummary]. (n.d.). Retrieved February 10, 2018,
from National Cancer Institute website: https://www.cancer.gov/about-cancer/
treatment/side-effects/sleep-disorders-pdq#section/_3

Sonima Guided Meditations: Learn to Relax Your Mind & Focus With
Calmness. (n.d.). Retrieved July 23, 2019, from Sonima website:
https://www.sonima.com/meditation/guided-meditations-meditation/

Wildmind Buddhist Meditation Homepage. (n.d.). Retrieved February 20, 2018,
from Wildmind Buddhist Meditation website: https://www.wildmind.org

Academic Research Articles

Abelson, J. L., Erickson, T. M., Mayer, S. E., Crocker, J., Briggs, H., Lopez-Duran,
N. L., & Liberzon, I. (2014). Brief cognitive intervention can modulate
neuroendocrine stress responses to the Trier Social Stress Test: Buffering effects
of a compassionate goal orientation. *Psychoneuroendocrinology, 44*, 60–70.
https://doi.org/10.1016/j.psyneuen.2014.02.016

Abrahams, H. J. G., Gielissen, M. F. M., Schmits, I. C., Verhagen, C. a. H. H. V.
M., Rovers, M. M., & Knoop, H. (2016). Risk factors, prevalence, and course
of severe fatigue after breast cancer treatment: A meta-analysis involving 12 327
breast cancer survivors. *Annals of Oncology: Official Journal of the European Society
for Medical Oncology, 27*(6), 965–974. https://doi.org/10.1093/annonc/mdw099

Albers, J. W., Chaudhry, V., Cavaletti, G., & Donehower, R. C. (2014).
Interventions for preventing neuropathy caused by cisplatin and related

compounds. *The Cochrane Database of Systematic Reviews*, (3), CD005228. https://doi.org/10.1002/14651858.CD005228.pub4

Amara, S. (2008). Oral glutamine for the prevention of chemotherapy-induced peripheral neuropathy. *The Annals of Pharmacotherapy*, *42*(10), 1481–1485. https://doi.org/10.1345/aph.1L179

Andreyev, J., Ross, P., Donnellan, C., Lennan, E., Leonard, P., Waters, C., ... Ferry, D. (2014). Guidance on the management of diarrhoea during cancer chemotherapy. *The Lancet. Oncology*, *15*(10), e447-460. https://doi.org/10.1016/S1470-2045(14)70006-3

Ansari, M., Porouhan, P., Mohammadianpanah, M., Omidvari, S., Mosalaei, A., Ahmadloo, N., ... Hamedi, S. H. (2016). Efficacy of Ginger in Control of Chemotherapy Induced Nausea and Vomiting in Breast Cancer Patients Receiving Doxorubicin-Based Chemotherapy. *Asian Pacific Journal of Cancer Prevention: APJCP*, *17*(8), 3877–3880.

Areti, A., Yerra, V. G., Naidu, V., & Kumar, A. (2014). Oxidative stress and nerve damage: Role in chemotherapy induced peripheral neuropathy. *Redox Biology*, *2*, 289–295. https://doi.org/10.1016/j.redox.2014.01.006

Aziz, M. T., Good, B. L., & Lowe, D. K. (2014). Serotonin-norepinephrine reuptake inhibitors for the management of chemotherapy-induced peripheral neuropathy. *The Annals of Pharmacotherapy*, *48*(5), 626–632. https://doi.org/10.1177/1060028014525033

Badowski, M. E. (2017). A review of oral cannabinoids and medical marijuana for the treatment of chemotherapy-induced nausea and vomiting: A focus on pharmacokinetic variability and pharmacodynamics. *Cancer Chemotherapy and Pharmacology*, *80*(3), 441–449. https://doi.org/10.1007/s00280-017-3387-5

Bailey, T. G., Cable, N. T., Aziz, N., Dobson, R., Sprung, V. S., Low, D. A., & Jones, H. (2016). Exercise training reduces the frequency of menopausal hot flushes by improving thermoregulatory control. *Menopause (New York, N.Y.)*, *23*(7), 708–718. https://doi.org/10.1097/GME.0000000000000625

Belcaro, G., Hosoi, M., Pellegrini, L., Appendino, G., Ippolito, E., Ricci, A., ... Togni, S. (2014). A controlled study of a lecithinized delivery system of curcumin (Meriva®) to alleviate the adverse effects of cancer treatment. *Phytotherapy Research: PTR*, *28*(3), 444–450. https://doi.org/10.1002/ptr.5014

Black, D. S., & Slavich, G. M. (2016). Mindfulness meditation and the immune system: A systematic review of randomized controlled trials. *Annals of the New York Academy of Sciences*, *1373*(1), 13–24. https://doi.org/10.1111/nyas.12998

Bossi, P., Cortinovis, D., Fatigoni, S., Cossu Rocca, M., Fabi, A., Seminara, P., ... Roila, F. (2017). A randomized, double-blind, placebo-controlled, multicenter study of a ginger extract in the management of chemotherapy-induced nausea and vomiting (CINV) in patients receiving high-dose cisplatin. *Annals of Oncology: Official Journal of the European Society for Medical Oncology, 28*(10), 2547–2551. https://doi.org/10.1093/annonc/mdx315

Bower, J. E., Crosswell, A. D., Stanton, A. L., Crespi, C. M., Winston, D., Arevalo, J., ... Ganz, P. A. (2015). Mindfulness meditation for younger breast cancer survivors: A randomized controlled trial. *Cancer, 121*(8), 1231–1240. https://doi.org/10.1002/cncr.29194

Brami, C., Bao, T., & Deng, G. (2016). Natural Products and Complementary Therapies for Chemotherapy-Induced Peripheral Neuropathy: A Systematic Review. *Critical Reviews in Oncology/Hematology, 98*, 325–334. https://doi.org/10.1016/j.critrevonc.2015.11.014

Brosschot, J. F., Verkuil, B., & Thayer, J. F. (2017). Exposed to events that never happen: Generalized unsafety, the default stress response, and prolonged autonomic activity. *Neuroscience and Biobehavioral Reviews, 74*(Pt B), 287–296. https://doi.org/10.1016/j.neubiorev.2016.07.019

Carlson, L. E., Doll, R., Stephen, J., Faris, P., Tamagawa, R., Drysdale, E., & Speca, M. (2013). Randomized controlled trial of Mindfulness-based cancer recovery versus supportive expressive group therapy for distressed survivors of breast cancer. *Journal of Clinical Oncology: Official Journal of the American Society of Clinical Oncology, 31*(25), 3119–3126. https://doi.org/10.1200/JCO.2012.47.5210

Carlson, L. E., Tamagawa, R., Stephen, J., Drysdale, E., Zhong, L., & Speca, M. (2016). Randomized-controlled trial of mindfulness-based cancer recovery versus supportive expressive group therapy among distressed breast cancer survivors (MINDSET): Long-term follow-up results. *Psycho-Oncology, 25*(7), 750–759. https://doi.org/10.1002/pon.4150

Chen, W. Y., Giobbie-Hurder, A., Gantman, K., Savoie, J., Scheib, R., Parker, L. M., & Schernhammer, E. S. (2014). A randomized, placebo-controlled trial of melatonin on breast cancer survivors: Impact on sleep, mood, and hot flashes. *Breast Cancer Research and Treatment, 145*(2), 381–388. https://doi.org/10.1007/s10549-014-2944-4

Chu, S. H., Lee, Y. J., Lee, E. S., Geng, Y., Wang, X. S., & Cleeland, C. S. (2015). Current use of drugs affecting the central nervous system for chemotherapy-induced peripheral neuropathy in cancer patients: A systematic review. *Supportive*

Care in Cancer: Official Journal of the Multinational Association of Supportive Care in Cancer, 23(2), 513–524. https://doi.org/10.1007/s00520-014-2408-8

Cohen, L. S., Joffe, H., Guthrie, K. A., Ensrud, K. E., Freeman, M., Carpenter, J. S., … Anderson, G. L. (2014). Efficacy of Omega-3 Treatment for Vasomotor Symptoms: A Randomized Controlled Trial. *Menopause (New York, N.Y.), 21*(4), 347–354. https://doi.org/10.1097/GME.0b013e31829e40b8

Cramer, H., Lauche, R., Klose, P., Lange, S., Langhorst, J., & Dobos, G. J. (2017). Yoga for improving health-related quality of life, mental health and cancer-related symptoms in women diagnosed with breast cancer. *The Cochrane Database of Systematic Reviews, 1*, CD010802. https://doi.org/10.1002/14651858.CD010802.pub2

Cramp, F., & Byron-Daniel, J. (2012). Exercise for the management of cancer-related fatigue in adults. *The Cochrane Database of Systematic Reviews, 11*, CD006145. https://doi.org/10.1002/14651858.CD006145.pub3

Crum, A. J., Akinola, M., Martin, A., & Fath, S. (2017). The role of stress mindset in shaping cognitive, emotional, and physiological responses to challenging and threatening stress. *Anxiety, Stress, and Coping, 30*(4), 379–395. https://doi.org/10.1080/10615806.2016.1275585

Daley, A., Stokes-Lampard, H., Thomas, A., & MacArthur, C. (2014). Exercise for vasomotor menopausal symptoms. In *Cochrane Database of Systematic Reviews*. https://doi.org/10.1002/14651858.CD006108.pub4

Davis, M. P. (2016). Cannabinoids for Symptom Management and Cancer Therapy: The Evidence. *Journal of the National Comprehensive Cancer Network: JNCCN, 14*(7), 915–922.

Davis, M. P., & Goforth, H. W. (2014). Long-term and short-term effects of insomnia in cancer and effective interventions. *Cancer Journal (Sudbury, Mass.), 20*(5), 330–344. https://doi.org/10.1097/PPO.0000000000000071

Del Fabbro, E., Dev, R., Hui, D., Palmer, L., & Bruera, E. (2013). Effects of melatonin on appetite and other symptoms in patients with advanced cancer and cachexia: A double-blind placebo-controlled trial. *Journal of Clinical Oncology: Official Journal of the American Society of Clinical Oncology, 31*(10), 1271–1276. https://doi.org/10.1200/JCO.2012.43.6766

Devin, J. L., Hill, M. M., Mourtzakis, M., Quadrilatero, J., Jenkins, D. G., & Skinner, T. L. (2019). Acute high intensity interval exercise reduces colon cancer cell growth. *The Journal of Physiology, 597*(8), 2177–2184. https://doi.org/10.1113/JP277648

Dimitrova, A., Murchison, C., & Oken, B. (2017). Acupuncture for the Treatment of Peripheral Neuropathy: A Systematic Review and Meta-Analysis. *Journal of Alternative and Complementary Medicine (New York, N.Y.)*, *23*(3), 164–179. https://doi.org/10.1089/acm.2016.0155

Dodin, S., Blanchet, C., Marc, I., Ernst, E., Wu, T., Vaillancourt, C., … Maunsell, E. (2013). Acupuncture for menopausal hot flushes. *The Cochrane Database of Systematic Reviews*, (7), CD007410. https://doi.org/10.1002/14651858.CD007410.pub2

Duran, M., Pérez, E., Abanades, S., Vidal, X., Saura, C., Majem, M., … Capellà, D. (2010). Preliminary efficacy and safety of an oromucosal standardized cannabis extract in chemotherapy-induced nausea and vomiting. *British Journal of Clinical Pharmacology*, *70*(5), 656–663. https://doi.org/10.1111/j.1365-2125.2010.03743.x

Elkins, G., Marcus, J., Stearns, V., Perfect, M., Rajab, M. H., Ruud, C., … Keith, T. (2008). Randomized Trial of a Hypnosis Intervention for Treatment of Hot Flashes Among Breast Cancer Survivors. *Journal of Clinical Oncology*, *26*(31), 5022–5026. https://doi.org/10.1200/JCO.2008.16.6389

Elkins, G. R., Fisher, W. I., Johnson, A. K., Carpenter, J. S., & Keith, T. Z. (2013). Clinical Hypnosis in the Treatment of Post-Menopausal Hot Flashes: A Randomized Controlled Trial. *Menopause (New York, N.Y.)*, *20*(3). https://doi.org/10.1097/GME.0b013e31826ce3ed

Eum, S., Choi, H.-D., Chang, M.-J., Choi, H.-C., Ko, Y.-J., Ahn, J.-S., … Lee, J.-Y. (2013). Protective effects of vitamin E on chemotherapy-induced peripheral neuropathy: A meta-analysis of randomized controlled trials. *International Journal for Vitamin and Nutrition Research. Internationale Zeitschrift Fur Vitamin- Und Ernahrungsforschung. Journal International De Vitaminologie Et De Nutrition*, *83*(2), 101–111. https://doi.org/10.1024/0300-9831/a000149

Freeman, M. P., Hibbeln, J. R., Silver, M., Hirschberg, A. M., Wang, B., Yule, A. M., … Cohen, L. S. (2011). Omega-3 fatty acids for major depressive disorder associated with the menopausal transition: A preliminary open trial. *Menopause (New York, N.Y.)*, *18*(3), 279–284. https://doi.org/10.1097/gme.0b013e3181f2ea2e

Freeman, M. P., Hirschberg, A. M., Wang, B., Petrillo, L. F., Connors, S., Regan, S., … Cohen, L. S. (2013). Duloxetine for major depressive disorder and daytime and nighttime hot flashes associated with the menopausal transition. *Maturitas*, *75*(2), 170–174. https://doi.org/10.1016/j.maturitas.2013.03.007

Fujiki, H., Watanabe, T., Sueoka, E., Rawangkan, A., & Suganuma, M. (2018). Cancer Prevention with Green Tea and Its Principal Constituent, EGCG: From

Early Investigations to Current Focus on Human Cancer Stem Cells. *Molecules and Cells, 41*(2), 73–82. https://doi.org/10.14348/molcells.2018.2227

Galley, H. F., McCormick, B., Wilson, K. L., Lowes, D. A., Colvin, L., & Torsney, C. (2017). Melatonin limits paclitaxel-induced mitochondrial dysfunction in vitro and protects against paclitaxel-induced neuropathic pain in the rat. *Journal of Pineal Research, 63*(4). https://doi.org/10.1111/jpi.12444

Garcia, M. K., Cohen, L., Spano, M., Spelman, A., Hashmi, Y., Chaoul, A., ... Lopez, G. (2016). Inpatient Acupuncture at a Major Cancer Center. *Integrative Cancer Therapies*, 1534735416685403. https://doi.org/10.1177/1534735416685403

George, M., Elias, A., & Shafiei, M. (2015). Insomnia in Cancer—Associations and Implications. *Asian Pacific Journal of Cancer Prevention: APJCP, 16*(15), 6711–6714.

Gibson, R. J., Keefe, D. M. K., Lalla, R. V., Bateman, E., Blijlevens, N., Fijlstra, M., ... Mucositis Study Group of the Multinational Association of Supportive Care in Cancer/International Society of Oral Oncology (MASCC/ISOO). (2013). Systematic review of agents for the management of gastrointestinal mucositis in cancer patients. *Supportive Care in Cancer: Official Journal of the Multinational Association of Supportive Care in Cancer, 21*(1), 313–326. https://doi.org/10.1007/s00520-012-1644-z

Goldstein, K. M., Coeytaux, R. R., Williams, J. W., Shepherd-Banigan, M., Goode, A. P., McDuffie, J. R., ... Wing, L. (2016). *Nonpharmacologic Treatments for Menopause-Associated Vasomotor Symptoms*. Retrieved from http://www.ncbi.nlm.nih.gov/books/NBK447618/

Greenlee, H., DuPont-Reyes, M. J., Balneaves, L. G., Carlson, L. E., Cohen, M. R., Deng, G., ... Tripathy, D. (2017). Clinical practice guidelines on the evidence-based use of integrative therapies during and after breast cancer treatment. *CA: A Cancer Journal for Clinicians, 67*(3), 194–232. https://doi.org/10.3322/caac.21397

Gul, K., Mehmet, K., & Meryem, A. (2016). The effects of oral glutamine on clinical and survival outcomes of non-small cell lung cancer patients treated with chemoradiotherapy. *Clinical Nutrition (Edinburgh, Scotland)*. https://doi.org/10.1016/j.clnu.2016.06.012

Guo, Y., Jones, D., Palmer, J. L., Forman, A., Dakhil, S. R., Velasco, M. R., ... Fisch, M. J. (2014). Oral alpha-lipoic acid to prevent chemotherapy-induced peripheral neuropathy: A randomized, double-blind, placebo-controlled trial. *Supportive Care in Cancer: Official Journal of the Multinational Association of Supportive Care in Cancer, 22*(5), 1223–1231. https://doi.org/10.1007/s00520-013-2075-1

Guthrie, K. A., LaCroix, A. Z., Ensrud, K. E., Joffe, H., Newton, K. M., Reed, S. D., … Anderson, G. L. (2015). Pooled Analysis of Six Pharmacologic and Nonpharmacologic Interventions for Vasomotor Symptoms. *Obstetrics and Gynecology, 126*(2), 413–422. https://doi.org/10.1097/AOG.0000000000000927

Hansen, M. V., Andersen, L. T., Madsen, M. T., Hageman, I., Rasmussen, L. S., Bokmand, S., … Gögenur, I. (2014). Effect of melatonin on depressive symptoms and anxiety in patients undergoing breast cancer surgery: A randomized, double-blind, placebo-controlled trial. *Breast Cancer Research and Treatment, 145*(3), 683–695. https://doi.org/10.1007/s10549-014-2962-2

Hershman, D. L., Lacchetti, C., Dworkin, R. H., Lavoie Smith, E. M., Bleeker, J., Cavaletti, G., … American Society of Clinical Oncology. (2014a). Prevention and management of chemotherapy-induced peripheral neuropathy in survivors of adult cancers: American Society of Clinical Oncology clinical practice guideline. *Journal of Clinical Oncology: Official Journal of the American Society of Clinical Oncology, 32*(18), 1941–1967. https://doi.org/10.1200/JCO.2013.54.0914

Hershman, D. L., Lacchetti, C., Dworkin, R. H., Lavoie Smith, E. M., Bleeker, J., Cavaletti, G., … American Society of Clinical Oncology. (2014b). Prevention and management of chemotherapy-induced peripheral neuropathy in survivors of adult cancers: American Society of Clinical Oncology clinical practice guideline. *Journal of Clinical Oncology: Official Journal of the American Society of Clinical Oncology, 32*(18), 1941–1967. https://doi.org/10.1200/JCO.2013.54.0914

Hilfiker, R., Meichtry, A., Eicher, M., Nilsson, B. L., Knols, R. H., Verra, M. L., & Taeymans, J. (2017). Exercise and other non-pharmaceutical interventions for cancer-related fatigue in patients during or after cancer treatment: A systematic review incorporating an indirect-comparisons meta-analysis. *Br J Sports Med*, bjsports-2016-096422. https://doi.org/10.1136/bjsports-2016-096422

Hill, D. A., Crider, M., & Hill, S. R. (2016). Hormone Therapy and Other Treatments for Symptoms of Menopause. *American Family Physician, 94*(11), 884–889.

Innominato, P. F., Lim, A. S., Palesh, O., Clemons, M., Trudeau, M., Eisen, A., … Bjarnason, G. A. (2016). The effect of melatonin on sleep and quality of life in patients with advanced breast cancer. *Supportive Care in Cancer: Official Journal of the Multinational Association of Supportive Care in Cancer, 24*(3), 1097–1105. https://doi.org/10.1007/s00520-015-2883-6

Irwin, M. R., Olmstead, R., Carrillo, C., Sadeghi, N., Nicassio, P., Ganz, P. A., & Bower, J. E. (2017). Tai Chi Compared With Cognitive Behavioral Therapy for the Treatment of Insomnia in Survivors of Breast Cancer: A Randomized,

Partially Blinded, Noninferiority Trial. *Journal of Clinical Oncology: Official Journal of the American Society of Clinical Oncology, 35*(23), 2656–2665. https://doi.org/10.1200/JCO.2016.71.0285

Jamieson, J. P., Crum, A. J., Goyer, J. P., Marotta, M. E., & Akinola, M. (2018). Optimizing stress responses with reappraisal and mindset interventions: An integrated model. *Anxiety, Stress, and Coping, 31*(3), 245–261. https://doi.org/10.1080/10615806.2018.1442615

Johns, C., Seav, S. M., Dominick, S. A., Gorman, J. R., Li, H., Natarajan, L., … Irene Su, H. (2016). Informing hot flash treatment decisions for breast cancer survivors: A systematic review of randomized trials comparing active interventions. *Breast Cancer Research and Treatment, 156*(3), 415–426. https://doi.org/10.1007/s10549-016-3765-4

Jolfaie, N. R., Mirzaie, S., Ghiasvand, R., Askari, G., & Miraghajani, M. (2015). The effect of glutamine intake on complications of colorectal and colon cancer treatment: A systematic review. *Journal of Research in Medical Sciences: The Official Journal of Isfahan University of Medical Sciences, 20*(9), 910–918. https://doi.org/10.4103/1735-1995.170634

Kerckhove, N., Collin, A., Condé, S., Chaleteix, C., Pezet, D., & Balayssac, D. (2017). Long-Term Effects, Pathophysiological Mechanisms, and Risk Factors of Chemotherapy-Induced Peripheral Neuropathies: A Comprehensive Literature Review. *Frontiers in Pharmacology, 8*, 86. https://doi.org/10.3389/fphar.2017.00086

Kim, P. Y., & Johnson, C. E. (2017). Chemotherapy-induced peripheral neuropathy: A review of recent findings. *Current Opinion in Anaesthesiology, 30*(5), 570–576. https://doi.org/10.1097/ACO.0000000000000500

Krizanova, O., Babula, P., & Pacak, K. (2016). Stress, catecholaminergic system and cancer. *Stress (Amsterdam, Netherlands), 19*(4), 419–428. https://doi.org/10.1080/10253890.2016.1203415

Krukowski, K., Nijboer, C. H., Huo, X., Kavelaars, A., & Heijnen, C. J. (2015). Prevention of chemotherapy-induced peripheral neuropathy by the small-molecule inhibitor pifithrin-μ. *Pain, 156*(11), 2184–2192. https://doi.org/10.1097/j.pain.0000000000000290

Kuriyama, A., & Endo, K. (2018). Goshajinkigan for prevention of chemotherapy-induced peripheral neuropathy: A systematic review and meta-analysis. *Supportive Care in Cancer: Official Journal of the Multinational Association of Supportive Care in Cancer, 26*(4), 1051–1059. https://doi.org/10.1007/s00520-017-4028-6

Lahart, I. M., Metsios, G. S., Nevill, A. M., & Carmichael, A. R. (2018). Physical activity for women with breast cancer after adjuvant therapy. *The Cochrane Database of Systematic Reviews, 1*, CD011292. https://doi.org/10.1002/14651858.CD011292.pub2

Lambertini, M., Del Mastro, L., Pescio, M. C., Andersen, C. Y., Azim, H. A., Peccatori, F. A., ... Anserini, P. (2016). Cancer and fertility preservation: International recommendations from an expert meeting. *BMC Medicine, 14*. https://doi.org/10.1186/s12916-015-0545-7

Leach, M. J., & Moore, V. (2012). Black cohosh (Cimicifuga spp.) for menopausal symptoms. *The Cochrane Database of Systematic Reviews, (9)*, CD007244. https://doi.org/10.1002/14651858.CD007244.pub2

Leal, A. D., Qin, R., Atherton, P. J., Haluska, P., Behrens, R. J., Tiber, C. H., ... Alliance for Clinical Trials in Oncology. (2014). North Central Cancer Treatment Group/Alliance trial N08CA-the use of glutathione for prevention of paclitaxel/carboplatin-induced peripheral neuropathy: A phase 3 randomized, double-blind, placebo-controlled study. *Cancer, 120*(12), 1890–1897. https://doi.org/10.1002/cncr.28654

L'Espérance, S., Frenette, S., Dionne, A., Dionne, J.-Y., & Comité de l'évolution des pratiques en oncologie (CEPO). (2013). Pharmacological and non-hormonal treatment of hot flashes in breast cancer survivors: CEPO review and recommendations. *Supportive Care in Cancer: Official Journal of the Multinational Association of Supportive Care in Cancer, 21*(5), 1461–1474. https://doi.org/10.1007/s00520-013-1732-8

Leung, H. W. C., & Chan, A. L. F. (2016). Glutamine in Alleviation of Radiation-Induced Severe Oral Mucositis: A Meta-Analysis. *Nutrition and Cancer, 68*(5), 734–742. https://doi.org/10.1080/01635581.2016.1159700

Li, M., Yue, G. G.-L., Tsui, S. K.-W., Fung, K.-P., & Lau, C. B.-S. (2018). Turmeric extract, with absorbable curcumin, has potent anti-metastatic effect in vitro and in vivo. *Phytomedicine: International Journal of Phytotherapy and Phytopharmacology, 46*, 131–141. https://doi.org/10.1016/j.phymed.2018.03.065

Li, X., Qin, Y., Liu, W., Zhou, X.-Y., Li, Y.-N., & Wang, L.-Y. (2018). Efficacy of Ginger in Ameliorating Acute and Delayed Chemotherapy-Induced Nausea and Vomiting Among Patients With Lung Cancer Receiving Cisplatin-Based Regimens: A Randomized Controlled Trial. *Integrative Cancer Therapies, 17*(3), 747–754. https://doi.org/10.1177/1534735417753541

Low Dog, T. (2005). Menopause: A review of botanical dietary supplements. *The American Journal of Medicine*, *118 Suppl 12B*, 98–108. https://doi.org/10.1016/j.amjmed.2005.09.044

Lu, Z., Moody, J., Marx, B. L., & Hammerstrom, T. (2017). Treatment of Chemotherapy-Induced Peripheral Neuropathy in Integrative Oncology: A Survey of Acupuncture and Oriental Medicine Practitioners. *Journal of Alternative and Complementary Medicine (New York, N.Y.)*, *23*(12), 964–970. https://doi.org/10.1089/acm.2017.0052

Lucas, M., Asselin, G., Mérette, C., Poulin, M.-J., & Dodin, S. (2009). Effects of ethyl-eicosapentaenoic acid omega-3 fatty acid supplementation on hot flashes and quality of life among middle-aged women: A double-blind, placebo-controlled, randomized clinical trial. *Menopause (New York, N.Y.)*, *16*(2), 357–366. https://doi.org/10.1097/gme.0b013e3181865386

Majithia, N., Loprinzi, C. L., & Smith, T. J. (2016). New Practical Approaches to Chemotherapy-Induced Neuropathic Pain: Prevention, Assessment, and Treatment. *Oncology (Williston Park, N.Y.)*, *30*(11), 1020–1029.

Maltser, S., Cristian, A., Silver, J. K., Morris, G. S., & Stout, N. L. (2017). A Focused Review of Safety Considerations in Cancer Rehabilitation. *PM&R*, *9*(9, Supplement 2), S415–S428. https://doi.org/10.1016/j.pmrj.2017.08.403

Mardas, M., Madry, R., & Stelmach-Mardas, M. (2017). Link between diet and chemotherapy related gastrointestinal side effects. *Contemporary Oncology (Poznan, Poland)*, *21*(2), 162–167. https://doi.org/10.5114/wo.2017.66896

Marx, W. M., Teleni, L., McCarthy, A. L., Vitetta, L., McKavanagh, D., Thomson, D., & Isenring, E. (2013a). Ginger (Zingiber officinale) and chemotherapy-induced nausea and vomiting: A systematic literature review. *Nutrition Reviews*, *71*(4), 245–254. https://doi.org/10.1111/nure.12016

Marx, W. M., Teleni, L., McCarthy, A. L., Vitetta, L., McKavanagh, D., Thomson, D., & Isenring, E. (2013b). Ginger (Zingiber officinale) and chemotherapy-induced nausea and vomiting: A systematic literature review. *Nutrition Reviews*, *71*(4), 245–254. https://doi.org/10.1111/nure.12016

McInnis, O. A., McQuaid, R. J., Matheson, K., & Anisman, H. (2017). Relations between plasma oxytocin, depressive symptoms and coping strategies in response to a stressor: The impact of social support. *Anxiety, Stress, and Coping*, *30*(5), 575–584. https://doi.org/10.1080/10615806.2017.1333604

Mishra, S. I., Scherer, R. W., Snyder, C., Geigle, P. M., Berlanstein, D. R., & Topaloglu, O. (2012a). Exercise interventions on health-related quality of life for people with cancer during active treatment. *The Cochrane Database of Systematic Reviews*, (8), CD008465. https://doi.org/10.1002/14651858.CD008465.pub2

Mishra, S. I., Scherer, R. W., Snyder, C., Geigle, P. M., Berlanstein, D. R., & Topaloglu, O. (2012b). Exercise interventions on health-related quality of life for people with cancer during active treatment. *The Cochrane Database of Systematic Reviews*, (8), CD008465. https://doi.org/10.1002/14651858.CD008465.pub2

Nangia, J., Wang, T., Osborne, C., Niravath, P., Otte, K., Papish, S., … Rimawi, M. (2017). Effect of a Scalp Cooling Device on Alopecia in Women Undergoing Chemotherapy for Breast Cancer: The SCALP Randomized Clinical Trial. *JAMA*, *317*(6), 596–605. https://doi.org/10.1001/jama.2016.20939

Nutrition and physical activity guidelines for cancer survivors. (2012). *CA: A Cancer Journal for Clinicians*, *62*(4), 275–276. https://doi.org/10.3322/caac.21146

Osório, C., Probert, T., Jones, E., Young, A. H., & Robbins, I. (2017). Adapting to Stress: Understanding the Neurobiology of Resilience. *Behavioral Medicine (Washington, D.C.)*, *43*(4), 307–322. https://doi.org/10.1080/08964289.2016.1170661

Ospina-Romero, M., Abdiwahab, E., Kobayashi, L., Filshtein, T., Brenowitz, W. D., Mayeda, E. R., & Glymour, M. M. (2019). Rate of Memory Change Before and After Cancer Diagnosis. *JAMA Network Open*, *2*(6), e196160–e196160. https://doi.org/10.1001/jamanetworkopen.2019.6160

Pachman, D. R., Barton, D. L., Swetz, K. M., & Loprinzi, C. L. (2012). Troublesome symptoms in cancer survivors: Fatigue, insomnia, neuropathy, and pain. *Journal of Clinical Oncology: Official Journal of the American Society of Clinical Oncology*, *30*(30), 3687–3696. https://doi.org/10.1200/JCO.2012.41.7238

Pachman, D. R., Dockter, T., Zekan, P. J., Fruth, B., Ruddy, K. J., Ta, L. E., … Loprinzi, C. L. (2017). A pilot study of minocycline for the prevention of paclitaxel-associated neuropathy: ACCRU study RU221408I. *Supportive Care in Cancer: Official Journal of the Multinational Association of Supportive Care in Cancer*, *25*(11), 3407–3416. https://doi.org/10.1007/s00520-017-3760-2

Parandavar, N., Abdali, K., Keshtgar, S., Emamghoreishi, M., & Amooee, S. (2014). The Effect of Melatonin on Climacteric Symptoms in Menopausal Women; A Double-Blind, Randomized Controlled, Clinical Trial. *Iranian Journal of Public Health*, *43*(10), 1405–1416.

Park, D., Yu, A., Metz, S. E., Tsukayama, E., Crum, A. J., & Duckworth, A. L. (2018). Beliefs About Stress Attenuate the Relation Among Adverse Life Events,

Perceived Distress, and Self-Control. *Child Development, 89*(6), 2059–2069. https://doi.org/10.1111/cdev.12946

Piccolo, J., & Kolesar, J. M. (2014). Prevention and treatment of chemotherapy-induced peripheral neuropathy. *American Journal of Health-System Pharmacy: AJHP: Official Journal of the American Society of Health-System Pharmacists, 71*(1), 19–25. https://doi.org/10.2146/ajhp130126

Prisciandaro, L. D., Geier, M. S., Butler, R. N., Cummins, A. G., & Howarth, G. S. (2011). Evidence supporting the use of probiotics for the prevention and treatment of chemotherapy-induced intestinal mucositis. *Critical Reviews in Food Science and Nutrition, 51*(3), 239–247. https://doi.org/10.1080/10408390903551747

Ramaswami, R., Villarreal, M. D., Pitta, D. M., Carpenter, J. S., Stebbing, J., & Kalesan, B. (2015). Venlafaxine in management of hot flashes in women with breast cancer: A systematic review and meta-analysis. *Breast Cancer Research and Treatment, 152*(2), 231–237. https://doi.org/10.1007/s10549-015-3465-5

Rethinking stress: The role of mindsets in determining the stress response. - PsycNET. (n.d.). Retrieved May 24, 2019, from https://psycnet.apa.org/record/2013-06053-001

Riley, P., Glenny, A.-M., Worthington, H. V., Littlewood, A., Clarkson, J. E., & McCabe, M. G. (2015). Interventions for preventing oral mucositis in patients with cancer receiving treatment: Oral cryotherapy. *The Cochrane Database of Systematic Reviews,* (12), CD011552. https://doi.org/10.1002/14651858.CD011552.pub2

Rithirangsriroj, K., Manchana, T., & Akkayagorn, L. (2015). Efficacy of acupuncture in prevention of delayed chemotherapy induced nausea and vomiting in gynecologic cancer patients. *Gynecologic Oncology, 136*(1), 82–86. https://doi.org/10.1016/j.ygyno.2014.10.025

Rossi, E., Di Stefano, M., Firenzuoli, F., Monechi, M. V., & Baccetti, S. (2017). Add-On Complementary Medicine in Cancer Care: Evidence in Literature and Experiences of Integration. *Medicines, 4*(1). https://doi.org/10.3390/medicines4010005

Rostock, M., Jaroslawski, K., Guethlin, C., Ludtke, R., Schröder, S., & Bartsch, H. H. (2013). Chemotherapy-induced peripheral neuropathy in cancer patients: A four-arm randomized trial on the effectiveness of electroacupuncture. *Evidence-Based Complementary and Alternative Medicine: ECAM, 2013,* 349653. https://doi.org/10.1155/2013/349653

Rotovnik Kozjek, N., Kompan, L., Soeters, P., Oblak, I., Mlakar Mastnak, D., Možina, B., … Velenik, V. (2011). Oral glutamine supplementation during preoperative radiochemotherapy in patients with rectal cancer: A randomised double blinded, placebo controlled pilot study. *Clinical Nutrition (Edinburgh, Scotland)*, *30*(5), 567–570. https://doi.org/10.1016/j.clnu.2011.06.003

Rouleau, C. R., Garland, S. N., & Carlson, L. E. (2015). The impact of mindfulness-based interventions on symptom burden, positive psychological outcomes, and biomarkers in cancer patients. *Cancer Management and Research*, *7*, 121–131. https://doi.org/10.2147/CMAR.S64165

Ruchlemer, R., Amit-Kohn, M., Raveh, D., & Hanuš, L. (2015). Inhaled medicinal cannabis and the immunocompromised patient. *Supportive Care in Cancer: Official Journal of the Multinational Association of Supportive Care in Cancer*, *23*(3), 819–822. https://doi.org/10.1007/s00520-014-2429-3

Rugo, H. S., Klein, P., Melin, S. A., Hurvitz, S. A., Melisko, M. E., Moore, A., … Cigler, T. (2017). Association Between Use of a Scalp Cooling Device and Alopecia After Chemotherapy for Breast Cancer. *JAMA*, *317*(6), 606–614. https://doi.org/10.1001/jama.2016.21038

Ryan, J. L., Heckler, C. E., Ling, M., Katz, A., Williams, J. P., Pentland, A. P., & Morrow, G. R. (2013). Curcumin for radiation dermatitis: A randomized, double-blind, placebo-controlled clinical trial of thirty breast cancer patients. *Radiation Research*, *180*(1), 34–43. https://doi.org/10.1667/RR3255.1

Sanada, K., Alda Díez, M., Salas Valero, M., Pérez-Yus, M. C., Demarzo, M. M. P., Montero-Marín, J., … García-Campayo, J. (2017). Effects of mindfulness-based interventions on biomarkers in healthy and cancer populations: A systematic review. *BMC Complementary and Alternative Medicine*, *17*(1), 125. https://doi.org/10.1186/s12906-017-1638-y

Sarkar, D. K., & Zhang, C. (2013). Beta-endorphin neuron regulates stress response and innate immunity to prevent breast cancer growth and progression. *Vitamins and Hormones*, *93*, 263–276. https://doi.org/10.1016/B978-0-12-416673-8.00011-3

Sato, J., Mori, M., Nihei, S., Kumagai, M., Takeuchi, S., Kashiwaba, M., & Kudo, K. (2016). The effectiveness of regional cooling for paclitaxel-induced peripheral neuropathy. *Journal of Pharmaceutical Health Care and Sciences*, *2*, 33. https://doi.org/10.1186/s40780-016-0067-2

Sayles, C., Hickerson, S. C., Bhat, R. R., Hall, J., Garey, K. W., & Trivedi, M. V. (2016). Oral Glutamine in Preventing Treatment-Related Mucositis in Adult

Patients With Cancer: A Systematic Review. *Nutrition in Clinical Practice: Official Publication of the American Society for Parenteral and Enteral Nutrition, 31*(2), 171–179. https://doi.org/10.1177/0884533615611857

Schellekens, M. P. J., Tamagawa, R., Labelle, L. E., Speca, M., Stephen, J., Drysdale, E., ... Carlson, L. E. (2017). Mindfulness-Based Cancer Recovery (MBCR) versus Supportive Expressive Group Therapy (SET) for distressed breast cancer survivors: Evaluating mindfulness and social support as mediators. *Journal of Behavioral Medicine, 40*(3), 414–422. https://doi.org/10.1007/s10865-016-9799-6

Schloss, J., & Colosimo, M. (2017). B Vitamin Complex and Chemotherapy-Induced Peripheral Neuropathy. *Current Oncology Reports, 19*(12), 76. https://doi.org/10.1007/s11912-017-0636-z

Schloss, J., Colosimo, M., & Vitetta, L. (2016). New Insights into Potential Prevention and Management Options for Chemotherapy-Induced Peripheral Neuropathy. *Asia-Pacific Journal of Oncology Nursing, 3*(1), 73–85. https://doi.org/10.4103/2347-5625.170977

Schloss, J., Colosimo, M., & Vitetta, L. (2017). Herbal medicines and chemotherapy induced peripheral neuropathy (CIPN): A critical literature review. *Critical Reviews in Food Science and Nutrition, 57*(6), 1107–1118. https://doi.org/10.1080/10408398.2014.889081

Schloss, J. M., Colosimo, M., Airey, C., Masci, P., Linnane, A. W., & Vitetta, L. (2017). A randomised, placebo-controlled trial assessing the efficacy of an oral B group vitamin in preventing the development of chemotherapy-induced peripheral neuropathy (CIPN). *Supportive Care in Cancer: Official Journal of the Multinational Association of Supportive Care in Cancer, 25*(1), 195–204. https://doi.org/10.1007/s00520-016-3404-y

Schloss, J. M., Colosimo, M., Airey, C., Masci, P. P., Linnane, A. W., & Vitetta, L. (2013). Nutraceuticals and chemotherapy induced peripheral neuropathy (CIPN): A systematic review. *Clinical Nutrition (Edinburgh, Scotland), 32*(6), 888–893. https://doi.org/10.1016/j.clnu.2013.04.007

Sideras, K., & Loprinzi, C. L. (2010). Nonhormonal Management of Hot Flashes for Women on Risk Reduction Therapy. *Journal of the National Comprehensive Cancer Network: JNCCN, 8*(10), 1171–1179.

Smith, L. A., Azariah, F., Lavender, V. T. C., Stoner, N. S., & Bettiol, S. (2015). Cannabinoids for nausea and vomiting in adults with cancer receiving chemotherapy. *The Cochrane Database of Systematic Reviews*, (11), CD009464. https://doi.org/10.1002/14651858.CD009464.pub2

Stobäus, N., Müller, M. J., Küpferling, S., Schulzke, J.-D., & Norman, K. (2015). Low Recent Protein Intake Predicts Cancer-Related Fatigue and Increased Mortality in Patients with Advanced Tumor Disease Undergoing Chemotherapy. *Nutrition and Cancer, 67*(5), 818–824. https://doi.org/10.1080/01635581.2015.1040520

Sun, Y., Shu, Y., Liu, B., Liu, P., Wu, C., Zheng, R., … Yao, Y. (2016). A prospective study to evaluate the efficacy and safety of oral acetyl-L-carnitine for the treatment of chemotherapy-induced peripheral neuropathy. *Experimental and Therapeutic Medicine, 12*(6), 4017–4024. https://doi.org/10.3892/etm.2016.3871

Sundar, R., Bandla, A., Tan, S. S. H., Liao, L.-D., Kumarakulasinghe, N. B., Jeyasekharan, A. D., Wilder-Smith, E. P. V. (2016). Limb Hypothermia for Preventing Paclitaxel-Induced Peripheral Neuropathy in Breast Cancer Patients: A Pilot Study. *Frontiers in Oncology, 6*, 274. https://doi.org/10.3389/fonc.2016.00274

Thamlikitkul, L., Srimuninnimit, V., Akewanlop, C., Ithimakin, S., Techawathanawanna, S., Korphaisarn, K., … Soparattanapaisarn, N. (2017). Efficacy of ginger for prophylaxis of chemotherapy-induced nausea and vomiting in breast cancer patients receiving adriamycin-cyclophosphamide regimen: A randomized, double-blind, placebo-controlled, crossover study. *Supportive Care in Cancer: Official Journal of the Multinational Association of Supportive Care in Cancer, 25*(2), 459–464. https://doi.org/10.1007/s00520-016-3423-8

Todaro, B. (2012). Cannabinoids in the treatment of chemotherapy-induced nausea and vomiting. *Journal of the National Comprehensive Cancer Network: JNCCN, 10*(4), 487–492.

Toivonen, K. I., Zernicke, K., & Carlson, L. E. (2017). Web-Based Mindfulness Interventions for People With Physical Health Conditions: Systematic Review. *Journal of Medical Internet Research, 19*(8), e303. https://doi.org/10.2196/jmir.7487

Tomlinson, D., Diorio, C., Beyene, J., & Sung, L. (2014). Effect of exercise on cancer-related fatigue: A meta-analysis. *American Journal of Physical Medicine & Rehabilitation, 93*(8), 675–686. https://doi.org/10.1097/PHM.0000000000000083

Topkan, E., Parlak, C., Topuk, S., & Pehlivan, B. (2012). Influence of oral glutamine supplementation on survival outcomes of patients treated with concurrent chemoradiotherapy for locally advanced non-small cell lung cancer. *BMC Cancer, 12*, 502. https://doi.org/10.1186/1471-2407-12-502

Touchefeu, Y., Montassier, E., Nieman, K., Gastinne, T., Potel, G., Bruley des Varannes, S., … de La Cochetière, M. F. (2014). Systematic review: The role of the gut microbiota in chemotherapy- or radiation-induced gastrointestinal mucositis - current evidence and potential clinical applications. *Alimentary Pharmacology & Therapeutics*, *40*(5), 409–421. https://doi.org/10.1111/apt.12878

Using Medical Cannabis in an Oncology Practice: Page 2 of 2 | Cancer Network | The Oncology Journal. (n.d.). Retrieved February 8, 2018, from http://www.cancernetwork.com/oncology-journal/ using-medical-cannabis-oncology-practice/page/0/1

Verma, V. (2016). Relationship and interactions of curcumin with radiation therapy. *World Journal of Clinical Oncology*, *7*(3), 275–283. https://doi.org/10.5306/wjco.v7.i3.275

Wang, W.-S., Lin, J.-K., Lin, T.-C., Chen, W.-S., Jiang, J.-K., Wang, H.-S., ... Chen, P.-M. (2007). Oral glutamine is effective for preventing oxaliplatin-induced neuropathy in colorectal cancer patients. *The Oncologist*, *12*(3), 312–319. https://doi.org/10.1634/theoncologist.12-3-312

Winocur, G., Johnston, I., & Castel, H. (2018). Chemotherapy and cognition: International cognition and cancer task force recommendations for harmonising preclinical research. *Cancer Treatment Reviews*, *69*, 72–83. https://doi.org/10.1016/j.ctrv.2018.05.017

Yi, J. C., & Syrjala, K. L. (2017). Anxiety and Depression in Cancer Survivors. *The Medical Clinics of North America*, *101*(6), 1099–1113. https://doi.org/10.1016/j.mcna.2017.06.00

Websites and Apps

6 Incredibly Useful Apps for Cancer Patients. (n.d.). Retrieved February 10, 2018, from TheSocialMedwork website: http://thesocialmedwork.com/blog/cancer-patient-tech-apps

10 Ways Exercise Helps During Cancer Treatment. (2017, February 9). Retrieved September 10, 2019, from American Physical Therapy Association website: https://choosept.com/resources/detail/ top-10-ways-exercise-helps-during-cancer-treatment

96 Percent Naturally Derived Ingredients—SkinActive—Garnier. (n.d.). Retrieved July 13, 2019, from https://www.garnierusa.com/shop-products/ skinactive/96-percent-naturally-derived-ingredients

The AARP 15-Minute Workout. May 16, 2016. (n.d.). Retrieved February 15, 2018, from AARP website: http://www.aarp.org/health/video-health/info-2016/the-aarp-15-minute-workout.html

About Us | Good Wishes. (n.d.). Retrieved June 27, 2019, from
http://www.goodwishesscarves.org/who-we-are/

Acupuncture Find a Practitioner Directory | NCCAOM. (n.d.). Retrieved February
8, 2018, from http://www.nccaom.org/find-a-practitioner-directory/

Acupuncture. (2011, December 1). Retrieved February 8, 2018, from NCCIH
website: https://nccih.nih.gov/health/acupuncture

ADA.gov homepage. (n.d.). Retrieved April 22, 2019, from https://www.ada.gov/

Alliance for Fertility Preservation | Fertility Preservation for
Cancer Patients. (n.d.-a). Retrieved July 25, 2019, from
https://www.allianceforfertilitypreservation.org/index.htm

American Cancer Society | Information and Resources about Cancer: Breast,
Colon, Lung, Prostate, Skin. (n.d.). Retrieved January 25, 2018, from
https://www.cancer.org

Best Cancer Blogs of 2019. (n.d.). Retrieved April 22, 2019, from
https://www.healthline.com/health/best-cancer-blogs-of-the-year#1

Breast Advocate® App. (n.d.). Retrieved August 7, 2019, from Breast Advocate® App
website: https://breastadvocateapp.com

Breathe2Relax | t2health. (n.d.). Retrieved June 4, 2017, from
http://t2health.dcoe.mil/apps/breathe2relax

Breathing Exercise: Three To Try | 4-7-8 Breath | Andrew Weil, M.D. (n.d.).
Retrieved February 11, 2018, from https://www.drweil.com/health-wellness/
body-mind-spirit/stress-anxiety/breathing-three-exercises/

Calm. (n.d.). Retrieved September 17, 2019, from https://www.calm.com

Cancer and Careers | The Top Resource for Working People With Cancer. (n.d.).
Retrieved September 4, 2019, from https://www.cancerandcareers.org/en

Cancer Legal Resource Center—a Disability Rights Legal Center site. (n.d.).
Retrieved April 22, 2019, from https://thedrlc.org/cancer/

Cancer patients given the royal treatment with stunning henna crowns.
(n.d.). Retrieved July 13, 2019, from Live Better With Cancer website:
https://cancer.livebetterwith.com/blogs/cancer/cancer-henna-crowns

Cancer Survival Toolbox. (n.d.). Retrieved February 10, 2018, from
NCCS - National Coalition for Cancer Survivorship website:
https://www.canceradvocacy.org/resources/cancer-survival-toolbox/

Cancercare.org Cancer, Support Groups, Counseling, Education, Publications, Financial Assistance. (n.d.). Retrieved January 25, 2018, from CancerCare website: https://www.cancercare.org/

Cancercenters.cancer.gov. (n.d.). Retrieved January 25, 2018, from https://cancercenters.cancer.gov/

Careers | Young Survival Coalition. (n.d.). Retrieved April 22, 2019, from Young Survival Coalition, Young women facing breast cancer together. website: https://www.youngsurvival.org/learn/living-with-breast-cancer/practical-concerns/careers

CareZone | Easily organize health information in one place. (n.d.). Retrieved February 10, 2018, from https://carezone.com/home

Caring and Comfort Wigs. (n.d.). Retrieved July 23, 2019, from https://www.caringandcomfort.com/

CaringBridge Personal Health Journals for Recovery, Cancer & More. (n.d.). Retrieved February 16, 2018, from CaringBridge website: https://www.caringbridge.org/

Chemo Cold Caps | Cold Cap Therapy. (n.d.). Retrieved February 9, 2018, from http://chemocoldcaps.com/

ChemoComfort. (n.d.). Retrieved June 16, 2019, from https://chemocomfort.org/

Chemotherapy | Fertility Risks from Treatment. (n.d.). Retrieved July 25, 2019, from https://www.allianceforfertilitypreservation.org/fertility-risks-from-treatment/chemotherapy

DoYogaWithMe.com Free Online Yoga Videos—Classes and Poses | DoYogaWithMe.com. (n.d.). Retrieved January 25, 2018, from https://www.doyogawithme.com/

Drake, E. (2015, August 26). 5 Things You May Not Know About Oncofertility. Retrieved February 10, 2018, from Huffington Post website: https://www.huffingtonpost.com/emily-drake/5-things-you-should-know-about-oncofertility_b_8037942.html

Eva | A mobile app for peer to peer cancer support. (n.d.-a). Retrieved July 27, 2019, from http://www.eva-app.co/

EWG. (n.d.). Healthy Living App (by EWG). Retrieved February 20, 2018, from https://www.ewg.org/apps

Exercise Builder—HEP2go—Build a HEP < Home Exercise Program> For Free. (n.d.). Retrieved September 10, 2019, from https://www.hep2go.com/index_b.php

Exercising at Home: Videos: NCHPAD - Building Inclusive Communities. (n.d.). Retrieved September 10, 2019, from National Center on Health, Physical Activity and Disability (NCHPAD) website: https://www.nchpad.org/Videos/PLwMObYmlSHaN0Pbu2xXymDUePlsTCsn7n

Exercising During Cancer Treatment. (n.d.). Retrieved February 15, 2018, from https://www.nccn.org/patients/resources/life_with_cancer/exercise.aspx

Family and Medical Leave Act—Wage and Hour Division (WHD)—U.S. Department of Labor. (n.d.). Retrieved April 22, 2019, from https://www.dol.gov/whd/fmla/index.htm

Foodsafety.gov. (n.d.). Recalls & Alerts. Retrieved February 19, 2018, from https://www.foodsafety.gov/recalls/index.html

For the Breast of Us. (n.d.). Retrieved June 26, 2019, from For the Breast of Us website: https://www.breastofus.com/

Free "Essentials of Cancer Exercise." (n.d.). Retrieved September 10, 2019, from Cancer Exercise Training Institute website: https://thecancerspecialist.com/free-essentials-of-cancer-exercise/

Free Guided Meditations—UCLA Mindful Awareness Research Center—Los Angeles, CA. (n.d.). Retrieved February 20, 2018, from http://marc.ucla.edu/mindful-meditations

Gaia—Conscious Media, Yoga & More. (n.d.). Retrieved January 25, 2018, from Gaia website: https://www.gaia.com

Gem Gem's Ginger Candy. (n.d.). Retrieved February 7, 2018, from http://www.gemgemsweet.com/about.en

Genetic Information Nondiscrimination Act of 2008. (n.d.). Retrieved April 22, 2019, from https://www.eeoc.gov/laws/statutes/gina.cfm

Gin Gins® Original Chewy Ginger Candy. (n.d.). Retrieved February 7, 2018, from https://gingerpeople.com/products/gin-gins-original-chewy-ginger-candy/

Ginger Aid®. (n.d.). Retrieved February 7, 2018, from Traditional Medicinals website: https://www.traditionalmedicinals.com/products/ginger-aid/

Ginger Honey Tea. (n.d.). Retrieved February 8, 2018, from Food Network website: https://www.foodnetwork.com/recipes/rachael-ray/ginger-honey-tea-recipe-1917101

Ginger Root Tea. (n.d.). Retrieved February 7, 2018, from http://www.buddhateas.com/ginger-root-tea.html

Glo | Unlimited access to yoga, meditation, and Pilates classes. Retrieved July 23, 2019, from https://www.glo.com/

GRYT Health: A Digital Health Company with a Social Purpose. (n.d.). Retrieved July 25, 2019, from GRYT Health website: https://grythealth.com/

Guide2chemo.com. (2014, March 4). Retrieved February 20, 2018, from http://guide2chemo.com/chemo-basics

Healthy_sleep.pdf. (n.d.). Retrieved from https://www.nhlbi.nih.gov/files/docs/public/sleep/healthy_sleep.pdf

Here For You—Thoughtful Care Packages for Life's Toughest Transitions. (n.d.). Retrieved April 22, 2019, from Here For You website: https://hereforyou.co/

How to appeal an insurance company decision. (n.d.). Retrieved February 8, 2018, from HealthCare.gov website: https://www.healthcare.gov/appeal-insurance-company-decision/appeals/

IHadCancer.com. (n.d.-a). Cancer Support Community for Peer to Peer Help |... Retrieved July 25, 2019, from https://www.ihadcancer.com/

Insight Timer Meditation Timer. Retrieved January 25, 2018, from https://insighttimer.com

Invisible Disabilities Association—IDA - Encourage | Educate | Connect | Invisible No More. (n.d.). Retrieved January 25, 2018, from Invisible Disabilities Association—IDA website: https://invisibledisabilities.org/

Johnson, J., & Alum, Y. S. C. (2016, July 11). 15 Ways You Can Help a Young Woman Diagnosed with Breast Cancer. Retrieved June 29, 2019, from Young Survival Coalition website: https://blog.youngsurvival. org/15-ways-you-can-help-a-young-woman-diagnosed-with-breast-cancer/

Kundalini Breathing Pranayam Techniques. (n.d.). Retrieved February 18, 2018, from 3HO - Happy, Healthy, Holy website: https://www.3ho.org/kundalini-yoga/pranayam/pranayam-techniques

Live Better With Cancer (UK). (n.d.). Retrieved February 20, 2018, from https://livebetterwith.com/

Living With App | This Is Living With Cancer | Official Site. (n.d.). Retrieved August 16, 2019, from https://www.thisislivingwithcancer.com/living-with-app

Livestrong. Retrieved September 18, 2019, from https://www.livestrong.org/we-can-help/livestrong-fertility

Look Good Feel Better. (n.d.). Retrieved January 25, 2018, from Look Good Feel Better website: http://lookgoodfeelbetter.org/

Mindful.org Meditation. (n.d.). Retrieved June 4, 2017, from https://www.mindful.org/meditation/

MoveforwardPT.com Cancer Page. (2017, February 1). Retrieved February 15, 2018, from American Physical Therapy Association website: https://www.moveforwardpt.com/SymptomsConditionsDetail.aspx?cid=256fdb5e-efde-44db-bbb3-ca2d56e68b50

Mrs.Mindfulness.com. (n.d.). Retrieved February 20, 2018, from Mrs. Mindfulness website: https://mrsmindfulness.com/

My Lifeline: Cancer support, free personal cancer patient websites and blogs, information about cancer treatment, and being a patient caregiver. (n.d.). Retrieved April 25, 2019, from MyLifeLine website: https://www.mylifeline.org/

National Cancer Institute. (n.d.). Retrieved January 25, 2018, from https://www.cancer.gov/

National Coalition for Cancer Survivorship (NCCS). (n.d.). Retrieved August 3, 2019, from NCCS - National Coalition for Cancer Survivorship website: https://www.canceradvocacy.org/

National Sleep Foundation—Sleep Research & Education. (n.d.). Retrieved February 10, 2018, from https://sleepfoundation.org/

Navigating Care. (n.d.). Retrieved February 16, 2018, from http://www.navigatingcare.com/patient/

NCCN - Evidence-Based Cancer Guidelines, Oncology Drug Compendium, Oncology Continuing Medical Education. (n.d.). Retrieved February 15, 2018, from https://www.nccn.org/

Nextdoor is the free private social network for your neighborhood community. (n.d.). Retrieved April 22, 2019, from Nextdoor.com website: https://nextdoor.com/

Oncolink. (n.d.). Retrieved February 10, 2018, from https://www.oncolink.org/

Open Heart Project. (n.d.). Retrieved February 20, 2018, from Susan Piver website: https://susanpiver.com/open-heart-project/

Our Story | The Cancer Journey. (n.d.). Retrieved May 21, 2019, from http://www.thecancerjourney.com/about/our-story/

PAN Foundation—Home. (n.d.). Retrieved September 3, 2019, from https://panfoundation.org/index.php/en/

Parker, M., & at 28, D. (2019, June 25). Cancer Ever AFTER: Monisha's Story | YSC Blog. Retrieved June 29, 2019, from Young Survival Coalition website: https://blog.youngsurvival.org/cancer-ever-after/

Patient Advocate Foundation. (n.d.). Retrieved February 8, 2018, from http://patientadvocate.org/

Paxman Scalp Cooling. (n.d.). Retrieved February 9, 2018, from Paxman USA website: https://www.paxmanusa.com

Penguin Cold Caps. (n.d.). Retrieved February 9, 2018, from Penguin Cold Caps website: https://penguincoldcaps.com/us/

Physical Activity and the Cancer Patient. (n.d.). Retrieved September 10, 2019, from https://www.cancer.org/treatment/survivorship-during-and-after-treatment/staying-active/physical-activity-and-the-cancer-patient.html

Pocket Cancer Care Guide. (n.d.). Retrieved February 10, 2018, from NCCS - National Coalition for Cancer Survivorship website: https://www.canceradvocacy.org/resources/pocket-care-guide/

Qigong Institute. (n.d.). Retrieved July 23, 2019, from https://www.qigonginstitute.org/

Rethink Breast Cancer. (2015, August 23). Retrieved February 9, 2018, from Rethink Breast Cancer website: https://rethinkbreastcancer.com/news/

Scalp Cooling System from Dignitana | Cold Caps | Chemotherapy Hair Loss. (n.d.-a). Retrieved February 9, 2018, from Dignicap website: https://dignicap.com/

Sleep Disorders [PdqCancerInfoSummary]. (n.d.). Retrieved February 10, 2018, from National Cancer Institute website: https://www.cancer.gov/about-cancer/treatment/side-effects/sleep-disorders-pdq#section/_3

Soluble Fiber Primer—Plus the Top Five Foods That Can Lower LDL Cholesterol. (n.d.). Retrieved February 9, 2018, from http://www.todaysdietitian.com/newarchives/120913p16.shtml

Sonima Guided Meditations: Learn to Relax Your Mind & Focus With Calmness. (n.d.-a). Retrieved July 23, 2019, from Sonima website: https://www.sonima.com/meditation/guided-meditations-meditation/

Sounds True. (n.d.). Retrieved January 25, 2018, from Sounds True website: https://www.soundstrue.com/store/

Tai Chi and Qi Gong for Health and Well-Being Video. (2012, January 6). Retrieved July 23, 2019, from NCCIH website: https://nccih.nih.gov/video/taichidvd-full

Tai Chi for Health Institute Dr. Paul Lam. (n.d.). Retrieved February 21, 2018, from Tai Chi for Health Institute website: https://taichiforhealthinstitute.org/what-is-tai-chi/

Talk to Someone: Triple Negative Breast Cancer. (n.d.). Retrieved June 26, 2019, from Kognito website: http://kognito.com/products/talk-to-someone-triple-negative-breast-cancer

Talking to Kids & Teens about Cancer | Cancer Support
    Community. (n.d.). Retrieved April 24, 2019, from
    https://www.cancersupportcommunity.org/talking-kids-teens-about-cancer

Teen Cancer America—Resources. (n.d.). Retrieved April 24, 2019, from Teen
    Cancer America website: https://teencanceramerica.org/news-resources/resources/

The Rapunzel Project® > Home. (n.d.). Retrieved February 9, 2018, from
    http://rapunzelproject.org/

The Ultimate High-Fiber Grocery List. (n.d.). Retrieved February 8, 2018, from
    https://www.webmd.com/cholesterol-management/features/fiber-groceries

Trader Joe's Homepage. (n.d.). Retrieved February 7, 2018, from
    https://www.traderjoes.com/

Triage Cancer. (2012, May 9). Retrieved August 3, 2019, from Triage Cancer web-
    site: https://triagecancer.org/

Understanding the stress response. Retrieved January 25, 2018,
    from Harvard Health Publishing, H. H. (n.d.). website:
    https://www.health.harvard.edu/staying-healthy/understanding-the-stress-response

Waking Up with Sam Harris—Discover your mind. (n.d.). Retrieved July 23, 2019,
    from Waking Up website: https://wakingup.com/

What is Tai Chi? Retrieved July 23, 2019, from Tai Chi for Health Institute website:
    https://taichiforhealthinstitute.org/what-is-tai-chi/

Wildmind Buddhist Meditation Homepage. (n.d.). Retrieved February 20, 2018,
    from Wildmind Buddhist Meditation website: https://www.wildmind.org

Wolin, K. Y., Schwartz, A. L., Matthews, C. E., Courneya, K. S., &
    Schmitz, K. H. (2012). Implementing the Exercise Guidelines for
    Cancer Survivors. *The Journal of Supportive Oncology*, *10*(5), 171–177.
    https://doi.org/10.1016/j.suponc.2012.02.001

Work and cancer. (n.d.). Retrieved September 4, 2019, from
    https://www.macmillan.org.uk/information-and-support/organising/work-and-cancer

Working with Cancer. (n.d.). Retrieved September 4, 2019, from
    https://www.workingwithcancer.co.uk/

Yoga Journal—Yoga Poses, Meditations, Sequences, and Free Classes.
    (n.d.). Retrieved July 23, 2019, from Yoga Journal website:
    https://www.yogajournal.com/

ACKNOWLEDGEMENTS

I am thankful for the help of so many people. My husband Bruno, whose love and level-headed support got the whole family through the writing and publishing process. Our boys, Bruno and Diego, who provided humor and motivation, and my entire extended family, who cheered me on. Shaghayegh Setayesh, who urged me to write the book in the first place, and Golbarg Karimkhanzand, who helped inspire it. My editor Janice Harper, who showed me the way and kept me on track.

I thank my many early readers: James R. Aist, Vivienne Armentrout, Patty and Mariano "Bean" Ayala, Melanie Burm, Heather Gilman Clay, Karen Cuellar, Michelle Figueroa, Michael Gonzalez, Christopher Lamott, Amy Lang MD, Bonnie Manion, Billie Marek MD, Trey Martinez, Kelly Montgomery, Wayne Moore, Laura Rocco, Keely Rodriguez, Kirstin Silberschlag, Kim Valle, Lou Wilmot, Carlene Yeager, Sheila Young and Rose Mary Zucker. I owe a special debt to my beta-readers for their heartfelt and specific feedback: Stephany Angelacos, Mari Bezuidenhout, Lara Bodary, Patricia Prijatel and Lecia Sequist, MD.

I am grateful to my medical team: Fitch Finnie, MD; Amy Lang, MD; Billie Marek, MD; Alex Miller, MD; Chet Nastala, MD; and the entire nursing and support staff at PRMA and the START Center for Cancer Care in San Antonio for caring for me throughout my cancer treatment. Your wonderful care was part of the inspiration for the book. Finally, I offer eternal gratitude to my family and friends who put their lives on hold to support me during my chemotherapy and cancer treatment. I literally would not be here otherwise.

ABOUT THE AUTHOR

Beverly A. Zavaleta, MD, is a board-certified family physician, cancer survivor and long-time advocate of patient education. After receiving her medical degree from Harvard Medical School, where she designed and implemented an asthma patient education program, she completed her residency training in family medicine at Christus Santa Rosa Hospital in San Antonio, Texas. In 2015, she was diagnosed with triple-negative breast cancer and underwent a grueling chemotherapy regimen. That experience, along with her experience as a doctor treating patients with cancer, led her to turn her attention to filling the gap in chemotherapy-focused patient education materials by writing *Braving Chemo*. Dr. Zavaleta practices as a primary care physician, and her health-related articles have appeared in the *Brownsville Herald* and on KevinMD. She lives in the Rio Grande Valley of South Texas with her husband, two sons and two dogs, and when not making a mess of her garden, she is reading or doing yoga. For bonus material, more chemotherapy tips and *Braving Chemo* updates, sign up at **https://www.BeverlyZavaletaMD.com** or follow her on Twitter and Instagram at @BZavaletaMD.

CPSIA information can be obtained
at www.ICGtesting.com
Printed in the USA
LVHW081323251120
672671LV00009B/25